Anastas, Lila

Your career in nursing

DATE DUE			
DEC 2 2 1998			
DEC 2 2 1998			
MAY 1 0 1999			
JUL 2 9 2003			
MAR 2 3 2004			
OCT 2 7 2014			
MAY 01 2017			

Your Career in Nursing

Lila Anastas, RN

Pub. No. 14-2216

National League for Nursing • New York

ISBN 0-88737-396-8

Second Edition

Manufactured in the United States of America

Preface to the First Edition

Your Career in Nursing is intended as a guide for persons interested in becoming a nurse, for students in formal nursing programs, for nurses returning to active professional service, and for nursing graduates (particularly baccalaureate graduates) who are exploring various career options.

Twenty-five years ago, when I was considering the profession of nursing, I would have found a career book such as this to be very helpful. I could have made a more informed choice had I known about personal aptitudes and abilities, the advantages and disadvantages of various educational programs, and the importance of on-the-job experience. If I were a young man, I would particularly have appreciated the information about men in nursing.

As a student in a baccalaureate nursing program, I would have liked to have had the facts and figures about the profession as well as information on licensing examinations and nursing organizations. Most important, I would have improved my sense of identity by learning about other members of my chosen profession, both those who take their place in history and those who serve as today's role models. In those confusing student days, I desperately wanted to know about nurses who were practicing in foreign lands or who were doing significant research or pursuing leadership positions. I wanted to know how they got from my place as a student to their esteemed places in nursing. The reader of this book will meet many nurses who openly shared their rich experiences. I, and they, hope that this will clear up some of the mystery for those practitioners who are to follow in their footsteps or even blaze new trails.

As a baccalaureate graduate, I would have found *Your Career in Nursing* particularly helpful as I examined the career options that were available to me. That was over twenty years ago, and with recent scientific and technological breakthroughs, expanding health services, and our aging population, there are literally hundreds of possibilities for today's nurse. Many of these are discussed in some detail in this book. Because the profession of nursing will continue to play an even more significant role in the future health care system, the challenges, the responsibilities, and the opportunities have never been greater than they are for today's nursing graduate.

When I started writing this book, I wanted, more than anything else, to bring nursing to life. I wanted the reader to meet some real nurses. I wanted the reader to sense the importance of a profession that is as old as humankind yet as dynamic and challenging as any in the health care system. To bring the profession to life, I talked with many nurses all across the country. With some, I shared their work place and walked by their sides as they went through a "typical" day. With others I had to depend on questionnaires or long telephone conversations. Out of this research came a book. Also out of my research came a tremendous pride in my fellow nurses. Their care and concern, brilliance and energy shone through. Some of these practitioners have served as role models for me as I have continued to learn and grow and to find my place in my profession. I hope they will do the same for you, the reader of this book.

Many generous people willingly gave their time and shared their thoughts with me. Because of space limitations, it is impossible to list all of them individually, but without their help, this book would not have been possible. I am particularly grateful to the staff of the National League for Nursing for their professional guidance and support.

All situations in this book are true and all nurses have allowed me to use their real names. In order to ensure their privacy, all patients' names have been changed.

I hope that the reader will find *Your Career in Nursing* to be a useful handbook, a convenient reference, and a source of inspiration.

Lila Anastas, RN

Preface

Nothing is as certain as change. Nursing is no exception to that rule.

Since I wrote the first edition of *Your Career in Nursing*, significant changes have occurred in health care and these in turn have affected the practice of nursing. Recent attempts to hold back hospital costs by instituting diagnostic related groups (DRGs), which also limit hospital stays, have caused drastic cuts in hospital budgets. As a result, hospitals have experienced severe nursing shortages and nurses find themselves caring for more seriously ill patients. Home health nurses and those employed in nursing homes face equal challenges as they care for an increasing number of patients who leave the hospital "quicker and sicker."

During this time of transition, there is an even greater need for well-educated, forward-thinking nurses who are willing to take positive action for the best interest of the health consumer.

In this second edition of *Your Career in Nursing*, I've focused on recent aspects of health care changes and their impact on the nursing profession. Discussion of DRGs, health maintenance organizations (HMOs), and other cost containment issues are as important to nursing as are recent technological advances. And the increased need for well-educated nurses can not be underestimated (the chapter on education reflects these new concerns). As health care becomes increasingly more complex, baccalaureate nurses and nurses with graduate degrees will be in even greater demand.

Finally, as nurses have become better educated, more confident and independent, new roles have emerged that could only be imagined ten years ago. Clinical specialists, nurse practitioners and now nurse entrepreneurs are the titles for today's nursing pioneers. Independent nurses who set up their own practices and do things the "nursing way" serve to strengthen all our ranks.

Once again, I owe a debt of gratitude to many individuals and organizations in helping me to update this book. I extend special thanks to the following educational programs: Orange County Community College (Middletown, New York); Lutheran General Hospital School of Nursing, Inc. (Park Ridge, Illinois); University of Michigan (Ann Arbor, Michigan); and University of California, San Francisco.

There is much to take pride in and much to look forward to. In many ways, there's never been a better time to be a nurse!

Lila Anastas, RN

Contents

Chapter 1   **What's It Like to Be a Nurse?**   **1**

NURSE-MIDWIFE   **1**
HOSPICE NURSE   **6**
LIFE FLIGHT NURSE   **10**
HOSPITAL STAFF NURSE   **14**

Chapter 2   **What Is a Nurse?**   **19**

HISTORY   **19**
   Florence Nightingale   **21**
   Nursing in the United States   **23**
DEFINITION OF NURSING   **27**
   Titles   **29**

Chapter 3   **Who Should Be a Nurse?**   **33**

INTERESTS, APTITUDES, AND ABILITIES   **33**
   Advantages of a Nursing Career   **36**
   Sources of Information   **38**
TODAY'S NURSE   **39**

Chapter 4   **Education**   **45**

WHAT PROGRAM OF STUDY?   **45**

PRACTICAL NURSING PROGRAMS   46
ASSOCIATE DEGREE PROGRAMS   47
DIPLOMA PROGRAMS   49
BACCALAUREATE PROGRAMS   54
MASTER'S PROGRAMS   58
CONTINUING YOUR EDUCATION   61
  Articulated Baccalaureate Programs   61
BECOMING AN RN: LICENSURE EXAMS   62
PUTTING YOUR BEST FOOT FORWARD   63
VOLUNTEER WORK   66

Chapter 5   The Real World of Nursing   69

FINDING A POSITION AS A GRADUATE
  NURSE   69
MAKING THE TRANSITION FROM STUDENT TO
  STAFF NURSE   71
KEEPING UP   73
  Continuing Education   73
  Career Mobility   73
  Non-Nurse College Graduates   74
NURSING ORGANIZATIONS   75
UNIONS   78

Chapter 6   Hospital Specialties   81

HOW A MODERN HOSPITAL IS SET UP   81
  The Nursing Department   82
  Ways of Organizing Nursing Care   85
  Hospital Shifts   86
HOSPITAL SPECIALTIES   87
  Emergency Room Nursing   87
  Medical Nursing   92
  Surgical Nursing   94
  Nurse Anesthetist   97
  Obstetrical Nursing   101
  Pediatric Nursing   103
  Other Specialties   105
THE NEW SPECIALTIES   106
  Critical-Care Nursing   106
  Burn Center   111

Dialysis Nurse   **114**
Oncology Nursing   **118**
Enterostomal Therapy   **120**
THE TREND TO SHORTER HOSPITAL
STAYS   **123**

Chapter 7   **Nonhospital Careers**   **127**

PSYCHIATRIC NURSING   **127**
REHABILITATION NURSING   **131**
Other Rehabilitation Units   **136**
NURSING HOMES   **136**
IN THE COMMUNITY   **140**
Office Nurse   **141**
Home Health Nurse   **144**
School Nurse   **150**
Occupational Health Nurse   **153**
AROUND THE WORLD   **155**
Military Nursing   **156**
Peace Corps   **160**
Public Health Service   **162**
Red Cross Nursing   **163**
Project HOPE   **164**
Other Opportunities   **165**

Chapter 8   **Teaching, Research, Administration, Law,**
Clinical Specialists, Communications   **167**

TEACHING   **167**
RESEARCH   **170**
ADMINISTRATION AND MANAGEMENT   **174**
NURSE ATTORNEY   **176**
CLINICAL SPECIALIST   **178**
COMMUNICATIONS   **181**

Chapter 9   **New Trends in Nursing**   **185**

THE ROLE OF THE MALE NURSE   **185**
NURSE PRACTITIONER—TODAY'S
PIONEER   **191**
Nurse-Midwives   **193**

Family Nurse Practitioner   **195**
Other Nurse Practitioners   **196**
Nurse Entrepreneurs   **197**
TOMORROW'S CHALLENGE   **201**
General Trends   **201**
Technology   **202**
Women and Nursing—New Images   **203**
The Nursing View   **203**

Appendix   **Additional Sources of Information**   **205**

INFORMATION ON EDUCATIONAL
   PROGRAMS   **205**
INFORMATION ON FINANCIAL
   ASSISTANCE   **206**
OTHER ORGANIZATIONS   **207**
TRAVEL AND MILITARY CAREERS   **211**
STATE BOARDS OF NURSING   **212**
   Separate State Boards of Practical Nursing   **215**

Glossary   **217**

Index   **223**

CHAPTER 1

What's It Like to Be a Nurse?

In recent years, there has been a consciousness raising among nurses, and many changes are now taking place in the profession. And in spite of some problems, there are many nurses who would never consider another profession. They are proud to be nurses and proud of the work they do. What exactly is that work like?

NURSE-MIDWIFE

Michael and Linda Lowe are expecting their first baby and have been under the care of the certified nurse-midwives (CNMs) at one of the thirteen San Diego-area perinatal clinics run by the University of California at San Diego Medical Center. The Lowes are young, have attended childbirth classes, and are hoping for a natural birth experience.

One summer night, labor begins, and when the contractions are regular and five minutes apart, Linda Lowe is admitted to the labor and delivery floor at UCSD Medical Center by Jan Hammond, CNM, who will be in charge of Mrs. Lowe's care. Ms. Hammond is one of the eight graduate nurse-midwives on staff. There are also six student nurse-midwives. Together they deliver about one-half the babies born at the Medical Center.[1]

---

[1]This description reflects nurse-midwifery practice in the state of California. In some states, a nurse-midwife may not deliver babies without a physician in attendance.

Linda and Michael are made comfortable in the alternate birth room—it is in this room that they would like to have their baby. There are a brass bed, pictures on the walls, and plants. But it's still a hospital room equipped with monitors and oxygen, and it is minutes away from even more sophisticated equipment.

It is 9:00 a.m. and labor is progressing well: the cervix, the opening of the birth canal, is stretched 8 cm and the baby is low in the pelvis. But the baby is large and there is a potential for difficulty. Mrs. Lowe is having trouble relaxing and has asked for something to relieve the pain. Ms. Hammond orders pain medication; in addition, an IV [2] is started in the patient's arm and oxygen is administered by a tube that is inserted into the patient's nose.

While making notes on Mrs. Lowe's chart, the nurse-midwife comments, "Patients usually want a totally natural birth experience, and that's our goal too. But, especially with a first baby, that isn't always possible. The Lowes' baby is large, and since the birth passage has not been tested before, labor may be long and there may be problems. When it's time for the baby to be born, we'll move Mrs. Lowe to the delivery room and I'll ask the doctor to stand by. The important thing here is that the mother be relaxed and that we have the best possible outcome for mother and baby. Sometimes it's just the right thing to give a little medication and get the patient back in control."

By 11:00 a.m., Linda Lowe appears very relaxed. She lies in bed on her left side supported with two blanket rolls, one at the small of her back and one between her knees. A monitor records the mother's contractions and the baby's heartbeat. The contractions are regular and of good strength, and the baby's heart rate is normal at 120. Mrs. Lowe rests between contractions. Mr. Lowe, dressed in a green scrub uniform, holds his wife's hand, strokes her forehead during the contractions, and offers encouragement. Ms. Hammond examines Mrs. Lowe and finds that her cervix is now 9 cm dilated. Mrs. Lowe asks, "How much longer?"

Ms. Hammond snaps off her rubber gloves as she replies: "We can't really think in terms of time but in terms of progress. And you're making great progress!" The nurse explains that the baby is going to be large and that, because this is Linda's first baby, it may take a little longer to move down the birth canal and under the pubic bone. "But the contractions are strong and you're doing very well."

Michael Lowe asks, "Are you sure the baby's in the right position?"

---

[2]See the Glossary at the back of this book for definitions of this and other technical nursing terms.

Ms. Hammond assures the couple that the baby is coming head first and is facing down. "Everything is as it should be. As soon as the opening of the cervix is stretched 10 cm, we can do some pushing with the contractions and help the baby to be born."

There's an easy rapport between the nurse and the couple. They know each other from clinic visits and the Lowes have confidence in the nurse-midwife's judgment. The nurse also knows what the Lowes expect from this birth. They had hoped for the event to move along more rapidly. Linda Lowe gazes at the clock and sighs.

The staff nurse assigned to Mrs. Lowe enters the room, and Ms. Hammond goes to the nurse's station to chart the patient's progress. Outside the room, Ms. Hammond explains, "Patience is probably the greatest virtue in obstetrics. When you get in the actual situation, of course, and parents and families are anxious—well, it's not easy to be patient."

Jan Hammond has worked in the Medical Center nurse-midwife program for two years. Before that, she worked for three years as an obstetrics/gynecology nurse practitioner with a group of doctors.[3] That was immediately after finishing the nurse practitioner program at the University of California at San Diego.

Far from being the stereotypical granny midwife, Jan Hammond is young, blond-haired, and attractive. She is soft-spoken and low-keyed. She has a warm personality and seems to like the work she does. "One of the challenges in working as a nurse-midwife is dealing with many different personalities and life-styles. I think that when people are growing up they imagine that the rest of the world is like their world, and of course that isn't true."

Ms. Hammond received her baccalaureate nursing education at California State College at Fresno. In her last two years there, she won a Navy scholarship. "I'd probably still be with the Navy today except that I developed a medical problem and had to leave the service."

In the labor room, Mrs. Lowe continues to make progress, and the nurse who has been observing her reports, "Mrs. Lowe said she feels a desire to push now."

Ms. Hammond checks her patient and finds that the cervix has stretched to 10 cm. Mr. and Mrs. Lowe know that a goal has been reached, and both smile at the news.

"You're now in Stage II labor, so with your next contraction, you can begin pushing. Remember in Lamaze classes how we did that?"

---

[3]See Chapter 2 for a description of the nurse practitioner role.

Ms. Hammond rolls up the head of the bed—"We'll let gravity help us out"—and reminds the Lowes of the breathing and mechanics of this stage of labor. Mr. Lowe is actively involved: he asks questions of the nurse-midwife and offers encouragement to his wife.

One midwife has described labor and delivery as "similar to running a twelve-mile race. The nurse-midwife is the manager. Dad is the coach, and Mom is the athlete." Some of that team action can be seen now. The atmosphere is positive and reassuring. From now until the moment of delivery, all attention is focused on the mother. Ms. Hammond sits at the foot of the bed. She observes, makes suggestions, and helps set the tone for all those present. As Linda Lowe pushes with the contractions, the staff nurse supports one of her knees and Michael Lowe supports the other.

"You're doing so well, Linda."

"You're not in this alone—we're all here with you."

"We know it's hard work but you're doing swell."

As more progress is made and a portion of the baby's head is visible (about the size of a half-dollar), another milestone is reached. "The baby is now under the pubic bone—let's get ready for a birthday party!"

Linda Lowe is transferred from the labor to the delivery room. Her husband, now wearing a special hat and static-free "booties," stays by her side. In the delivery room the pace quickens. Mrs. Lowe is placed on a special table with the head slightly elevated, her legs held apart and supported by low metal stirrups. She grips metal handles as the contractions continue. She is draped from the waist down in sterile material, and the birth area is cleansed. The overhead mirror is adjusted so that she can watch the birth.

Jan Hammond scrubs her hands and forearms and dresses in sterile gown and gloves. She has asked the attending physician to stand by during delivery because the baby is large. Now that monitors have been removed, the baby's heartbeat is checked with a portable electronic device.

Ms. Hammond has explained to the couple that an episiotomy will be necessary to allow more room for the baby to pass. "It's like making a gusset in a dress pattern—it'll prevent tearing as the baby comes out." The nurse-midwife gives the local anesthetic by injection and makes the cut.

The baby's forehead appears. "Linda, make this your longest push now—push past the burning and the hurt." Ms. Hammond helps the baby's birth by pulling gently downward. When the baby's face appears, the midwife suctions out the mouth with a rubber syringe, and after the shoulders have turned, the baby's body slides out in a gush of pink fluid.

"It's a boy!"

"What was that name again, Michael?"

The baby is placed in the waiting bassinet. Michael and Linda are smiling and laughing and crying. They touch their child and ask, still not quite believing, "Does he look normal?"

"He looks fine to me. Look at all that hair!"

Michael assists the staff nurse in cutting the cord. The baby screams and flails his arms and legs about. He receives an injection of Vitamin K ("to prevent internal bleeding") and eye drops ("to prevent infection").

Then the nurse and father give the baby his first bath and the infant is weighed. He tips the scale at 10 1/2 pounds: "That's close to a record for a first baby!"

The parents express their pride, happiness, and gratitude. Smiling eyes can be seen above the midwife's white mask. "Congratulations to you both!"

It has been ten minutes since the baby's birth. Ms. Hammond delivers the placenta and places it in a pan. That completes the third,

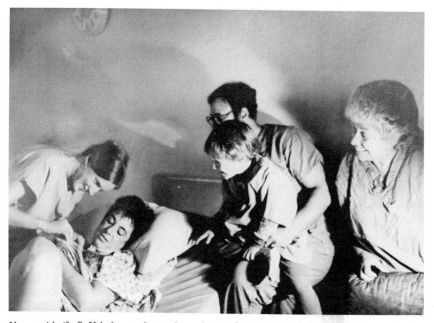

Nurse-midwife (left) helps mother with newborn infant while the father, son, and grandmother look on. *(Photo by Mariette Pathy Allen, Courtesy Maternity Center Association)*

or final, stage of labor. The midwife shows the placenta to Mrs. Lowe: "This is where the baby was staying—this is how he was nourished for nine months. Now I have to rub your lower belly. I'm sorry. I know it hurts, but that was a big baby and the uterus can bleed a lot. This will help tighten it up. You'll be breast feeding the baby, so that will help too."

Jan Hammond sews up the cut that was made before the baby's birth and continues talking with the new parents: "We could never have delivered that baby in bed. He was so big, I had to pull down to help deliver him."

The Lowe baby, wrapped in a warm blanket, is laid across his mother's chest—"So he can hear his mother's heartbeat"—and the lusty crying subsides for a moment.

It's a time of peace and tranquilitiy. Tiny baby fingers grip Michael Lowe's index finger. Husband and wife gaze at one another with the awe and excitement that new parents have experienced since the dawn of time. This triumphant moment is neither the beginning nor the ending of the couple's relationship with the nurse-midwife. But the drama of birth is the high point. And Jan Hammond, nurse-midwife, feels privileged to be a part of it.

HOSPICE NURSE

The car pulls up in front of a one-story stucco house in a suburban area of Southern California. Kirk Gresham, RN, gets out of his car and walks to the front door. He wears a white polo shirt and brown slacks and carries a small valise but no traditional nursing equipment. Kirk is the coordinator of patient care services for the Elizabeth Hospice in Escondido, California, and the greatest service he will bring to the family of Hank and Karen Bradley is his warm and caring presence.

Two months before, Hank Bradley received a death sentence from the medical profession. At age 49, he has inoperable lung cancer. He has completed a course of radiotherapy and is now receiving chemotherapy. In the judgment of his doctors, though, Hank Bradley will die within a year.

Nurse Gresham explains, "Mr. Bradley is unusual in several ways. First, his life expectancy is probably greater than six months, and usually we see patients with less than six months' life expectancy. But there was a real need—his wife very much wanted help—and the family is young. Most patients wait to call us until things are really bad. Fortunately, the Bradleys did not."

This is Kirk Gresham's second home contact with the family. The first, a two-hour assessment visit, was a month before. Since that time, Mr. Bradley has been in the hospital for treatment of dehydration and fluid imbalance.

Mrs. Bradley, a young attractive mother of two children, greets Nurse Gresham at the door. "I'm so glad you came. Hank's up in the chair today. Come in—."

Nurse Gresham is warm and friendly, but his tone is not falsely cheerful or light-hearted. The Bradleys are going through a difficult transition period that is heavy with fear and other strong emotions. Kirk greets and touches both patient and wife. He pulls up a chair close to Mr. Bradley as if to say, "I'm here to help—I'm not afraid and will not avoid you or this new issue in your life."

Hank, a tall, thin man dressed in a T-shirt and tennis shorts, reclines in a lounge chair. He smiles easily, and his face is gently furrowed with laugh lines. After the usual pleasantries, Kirk assesses his patient.

"Hank, you look 100 percent better today than the last time I saw you."

"I feel better too—at least 98 percent. You knew I was in the hospital a couple of weeks back, didn't you?"

"Yes—how *was* that ?"

"Well, I was sure I was going to die then. Just before I was admitted to the hospital—when I was in the doctor's office—I didn't know what was going on. I didn't know anybody. I was really out."

"Was that frightening to you?"

"No, not really. I look at it this way: when the time comes for me to die, I know a little of what it'll be like. I was close and it was very mellow. Not any pain—just a feeling of peace."

"So *that* fear is one you don't have to worry as much about—"

"Yeah. I was able to have a little of the experience beforehand."

"Like a practice run."

Bradley laughs, and, at the same time, seems to relax.

His wife, sitting across the room, curls up on the corner of the sofa and quietly contributes: "You know, we had our whole family here when Hank was in the hospital. It was beautiful—everybody together and caring. I think Hank's mother expected to see more of a change in her son. She was pleasantly surprised that he's still the same in many ways."

Hank and Karen continue to share the events and feelings in their lives. Kirk listens attentively, acknowledging their statements with a noncommittal "um-hum" or encouraging one line of thought with, "Can you tell me more about that?"

After the visit, Nurse Gresham comments, "It's hard to believe this is the same man who, when I first saw him, lay in his bed in extreme pain and was very reluctant to talk. The only thing he *would* talk about then was going back to work as a laborer. Now he sees this as an unrealistic plan. On that first visit, we discussed his illness and the course of therapy he would be taking, also symptoms and pain control. Then I explained about our program—that we could make available to him and his family a full range of services such as nursing care, home health aide services, social services and counseling, volunteer support and assistance, pain management consultation, nutritional education and bereavement counseling for the family for up to one year after the patient's death."

Nurse Gresham continues, "All of our services are coordinated by the hospice nurse with all medical decisions made by the patient's referring physician and reviewed weekly by the hospice team. This team, supervised by a medical director, also includes a physician (specially trained in the palliative approach encouraged by hospice), the patient's nurse, the social worker, counseling staff, the hospice chaplain, and any volunteers assigned to the case. It is the team's responsibility to assure that each hospice patient benefits from a truly holistic approach to his care. Right now we have 40 patients like Mr. Bradley in our caseload and another 120 families receiving bereavement follow-up. Nursing care and medical equipment are paid for through Medicare and other third party reimbursement while all other services are provided free of charge and supported by private grants and donations."

Hank Bradley pauses and takes sips of water from a glass. He tries to find a more comfortable position in his chair.

"You know, the other day I was sitting here and just feeling happy about all my blessings of life. The laundry was strung out on the back line, and the chickens and goats were in the yard. It was a clear day and I could see back to the hills. I saw how rich we are in the simple things of life. Maybe it was the first time I really saw it. I never took the time before."

"Do I hear some grief about lost time?"

"Definitely—especially time I didn't spend with my family. But I'm going to change that. I have a lot of time to sit and think now. And to say things I want to say. Like Karen here—she means the world to me. I owe her a great deal and I want her to know—."

Hank spontaneously gets up from his chair and moves to his wife's side. They embrace and share tears.

As the visit nears an end, Kirk talks briefly about relationships, past and present, and how important they are. He congratulates Karen on listening and supporting her husband. He congratulates Hank on being more in touch with his feelings. At no time during the visit has Kirk avoided the issues that are brought up. He doesn't change the subject or become preachy or judgmental. In simplest terms, Kirk is an active listener. But there's more to it than that—Kirk acts as a counselor, a friend, a social worker, and a nurse. It is hard to know where one role ends and another begins. His role as a hospice nurse is a unique one.

Hospice care is both the oldest and one of the newest specialties in nursing. The word *hospice* stems from the Latin for "host" or "guest." In the middle ages, hospice was a haven for weary travelers—a place for replenishment, refreshment, and care. The modern hospice was inspired by St. Christopher's Hospice in London, which was established in the mid-1960s. In the United States, they began in a more individualistic grass-roots fashion. Then in 1983 Medicare agreed to reimburse for specialized hospice care and established criteria for Medicare certification of hospice programs across the country. Since that time, many more hospices have been created nationwide and more insurers have included hospice services in their policies.

In this country, a hospice can be a program, a type of care, or a facility for the terminally ill and their families. As of this writing, Elizabeth Hospice is largely a community-based service, providing nursing care and respite inpatient beds through alliance with its local hospital district and home health agency. The program is currently awaiting the results of application for Medicare certification.

Kirk Gresham has been coordinator of patient care services at Elizabeth Hospice for one year, but his interest in death and dying goes back longer than that. "I was a student nurse when I had my first encounter with a dying patient. The man was comatose and very silently slipped away. It wasn't a dramatic physical event, but I felt that something big had happened and that it was an honor for me to be there. So I always had an interest and curiosity about death and sought out terminally ill patients as I worked in various hospitals. I attended conferences with Elizabeth Kubler-Ross and others in the field. I really feel that death is a social issue, and, because of the social avoidance, this has caused medical and emotional problems for patients and their families. The dehumanizing treatment of dying patients has led many to find 'something else.' That 'something else' is hospice care.

"Much of my working day is spent with a phone in one hand and patients' charts in front of me. It's an administrative job with the goal of coordinating the best type of care for the terminally ill patient. I call new referrals, physicians, agencies, and volunteers. I do assessment visits on new referrals and help the volunteer coordinator match patient and volunteer. Once a week I meet with the hospice team where we discuss and review decisions on all aspects of the patient's care. Twice a month the volunteers also meet separately with the volunteer coordinator to receive additional guidance and mutual support in the very sensitive and important work they do."

Lynette Goodman, RN, sets up the educational program for volunteers and arranges for classes at the local college or talks by community leaders. She teaches and gives talks in the community as well when the need arises. Her goal is for all persons to take a more humanistic approach to the terminally ill.

"As a hospital nurse, I saw a tremendous vacuum in the emotional care of surgical patients. Many nurses feel this frustration in traditional medical care—there's more emphasis on tasks than on emotional concerns. In hospice nursing, it's very rewarding to be able to share, at an intense level, the most critical, exciting, painful, and beautiful moments of a patient's life.

"But things do not always run smoothly. Sometimes patients don't want your help. And because this is such a new field, we're often the ones to make the guidelines—and to make the mistakes!"

What makes a good hospice nurse? Lynette and Kirk agree that the number-one criterion is that the nurse be nurturing and supportive. He or she should be a good listener and an emotional risk taker—that is, be able to jump in with his or her emotions and stay until the end. Experience as a medical and surgical staff nurse is helpful, and a personal or professional experience with a dying person is absolutely essential.

For Hank and Karen Bradley, the services of the Elizabeth Hospice mean living their lives as fully as possible, maintaining their dignity and humanness as death approaches, and having a friend and confidant throughout this time of transition.

LIFE FLIGHT NURSE

Late on a morning in August, Martha Bennett, RN, chief flight nurse of the Life Flight Team at UCSD Medical Center, had finished checking the flight equipment and was sitting in her office. She was reviewing a slide show to teach area fire fighters and police officers the how, when, and why of the helicopter medical service. Marti, as she is known by her co-workers, was dressed in the Life Flight uniform—navy blue twill jump suit and brown leather hiking boots. Marti was looking at slides on a viewer when a call came through on the communications hot line: "This is the sheriff's office. We need Life Flight to respond to Cuyamaca State Park ..."

Within five minutes, the pilot, another RN and Nurse Bennett are on the helipad located at the top of the Medical Center. The San Diego Flight program began in 1980 and has grown to include two fulltime helicopters plus a third on duty weekends. The copters are staffed by either two RNs or an RN and paramedic team. They are on call seven days a week, twenty-four hours a day, and serve primarily San Diego and Imperial counties. San Diego Life Flight averages 200 calls a month, 97 percent to the scene of the accident or illness.

Cuyamaca State Park is twenty minutes flying time from the hospital and is located in mountainous back country. On this Sunday, the termperature hovers around the 90° mark. The Life Flight helicopter lands, and the crew members grab their gear and rush to the scene. They make a quick assessment. A 50-year-old woman with a history of heart trouble is on vacation with her husband. While at the park, she was stricken with chest pain and difficulty in breathing. The patient took four tablets of the heart medicine that she carries with her, but it did not relieve her pain. While waiting for the Life Flight crew to arrive, the local volunteers took the patient's vital signs (blood pressure, pulse, and respiration) and gave her oxygen by mask.

The woman is sitting in the car in the parking lot. She complains of chest pain and is having trouble breathing. She is cyanotic (certain areas of her skin are bluish because there is insufficient oxygen in the blood). But her vital signs are within normal limits.

The Life Flight team works decisively as they remove the patient from the car and place her on a stretcher. A volunteer is asked to hold up a sheet to shield the woman from the noonday sun. The police have blocked off the road that leads to the parking lot. Another volunteer keeps away the curious bystanders.

Together the medical team hooks the patient up to the heart monitor. The patient shows PVCs (irregular heartbeats). An IV line is started, and medication is given to correct the abnormal heartbeat. The heart rate, which had been a normal 80, falls to the high 40s, and another medication is given to correct this problem. Because every second is important in Life Flight operations, the team's equipment is easily accessible and medications are color coded. The patient is connected to the Life Flight oxygen supply, and since the monitor still shows PVCs, Nurse Bennett runs ahead to the helicopter and puts together the equipment and medicine that will be necessary during flight.

The patient is carried to the helicopter and final plans are made to transport her to El Cajon Valley Hospital (the closest hospital with a helipad). The pilot explains to the patient's husband how to get to the hospital and cautions him to drive carefully. Meanwhile, the police and volunteers form a ring around the helicopter, and as soon as the area is free of people, the helicopter takes off. In the air, the medical team works in tight quarters. There are seats for the pilot and each member of the medical team, and space for two patient stretchers. The arrangement allows the medical team to maintain constant assessment of the patient and provide any additional care needed in flight. This is such an occasion. The monitor shows a more normal heart rate and Bennett administers morphine to relieve the patient's chest pain.

In a matter of minutes, the helicopter arrives at the hospital. Because the crew has radioed ahead, the hospital is awaiting the patient's arrival. She is transported to the cardiac care unit and the crew reports to the personnel there. Because of the prompt stabilization of the patient's condition by the Life Flight team, the patient's outlook for recovery is good.

While the crew is reloading for the return flight, a standby call comes through on the radio. The helicopter is refueled. The call becomes official. Next stop: Warner Springs.

Located sixty miles northeast of San Diego, Warner Springs is a dry, remote area famous for its warm springs. On this summer day, a young man and woman were riding together on a motorcycle at high speed along a narrow, twisting road. They skidded on a curve and went down on the left side of the road. The accident happened near the Naval Survival Center, and the couple was transported there by the police. The doctor assigned to the Center has already started an IV on the man.

When the helicopter lands, the crew goes to the aid of the two victims. The 26-year-old man was unconscious after the accident but is now awake, although not alert. He complains of abdominal and neck pain and multiple scratches and bruises on the left side of his body and a possible fracture of his left arm. His blood pressure is low, so the crew puts antishock trousers on him. These are a trouserlike piece of equipment that can be pumped up with air in order to apply pressure to the lower extremities, thus improving blood flow to the upper part of the body.

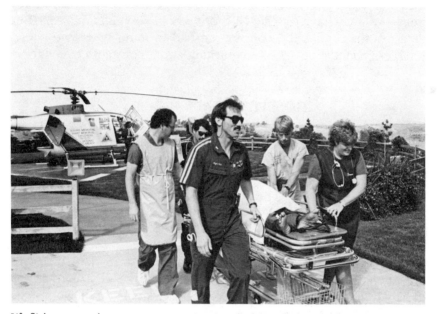

Life-flight nurse and crew transport a patient into the hospital. *(Courtesy Scripps Memorial Hospital)*

The other passenger on the motorcycle was a 19-year-old woman. Her vital signs are stable and she is completely conscious and alert. She has an open fracture of her left leg and a possible closed fracture of her left arm. She also has multiple scratches and bruises.

When the two patients are stabilized, they are moved onto backboards and stretchers and loaded in the helicopter for transport to Palomar Hospital, the nearest trauma center.

After returning to the Medical Center, Nurse Bennett removes all the equipment from the helicopter, puts in the duplicate backup equipment, and begins restocking her supplies. She can get back to her slide show later. Another call could come at any time.

Nurse Bennett is one of twenty-one nurses who work on Life Flight (seventeen are full-time, four are part-time). All have had previous emergency room experience and enjoy the challenge of this new kind of emergency care. The nurses work twelve-hour shifts.

Another flight nurse on duty summed up: "The work is hard but gratifying. When you're in the field you have to be innovative and creative. You don't have the backup equipment and personnel that the emergency room provides. In the air, you have to be aware of body changes at high altitudes. And you have to understand certain aviation regulations and safety factors. Also, we can get into some pretty rough areas—we may have to scale cliffs or work in very tight quarters. But it's a job that fulfills the concept we had in mind when we chose emergency medicine—it's very exciting and a constant challenge!"

HOSPITAL STAFF NURSE

Not all nursing care is given in large medical centers, and not all nurses are involved in such glamorous assignments as Life Flight or in such innovative fields as hospice nursing.

The life blood of any general hospital is the staff nurse. Day in and day out, this nurse gives important routine care to her patients. The pace may be slower in a smaller hospital than in a large medical center, but the challenge is just as great.

Sally Lessicka is a medical nurse at Pioneer's Memorial Hospital in Brawley, California. Located 120 miles east of San Diego in the Imperial Valley desert, the seventy-eight bed general hospital serves a mostly rural farming community whose population ebbs and flows with the movements of migrant workers and winter tourists. Because the town is located near the Mexican border, over half the population is Spanish speaking.

Sally Lessicka started her nursing career after her four children were grown, and she has assumed more and more responsibility since she became an RN in 1976. She is now supervisor of the hospital's medical unit.

"When I was a student in the associate degree program, I wanted more on-the-job experience, so I worked part-time as a nursing assistant at Pioneer's. I worked in all the departments and learned a great deal about being a hospital nurse. I learned a lot as a student, too, but it was different. In school, you worry about grades—in the work situation, you worry about your patients."

Most staff nurses at Pioneer's work eight-hour shifts. Ms. Lessicka punches in at 6:45 a.m. to start the day shift. She winds her way through brightly colored corridors and takes the stairs to the second floor. Besides the medical service, patients recuperating from surgery are on this floor. There's also the five-bed intensive-care unit, obstetrics, the newborn nursery, pediatrics (children's ward), and psychiatry. There are twenty-four beds on the medical wing, but there is room for overflow, and the number of patients changes frequently. The majority of the patients are elderly.

As a working supervisor, Ms. Lessicka is in charge of the unit, and her staff today consists of three RNs, one LVN (licensed vocational nurse), and two aides. (On evening and night shifts, there are fewer nurses and aides on staff.) The whole medical nursing staff congregates in the conference room for morning report. "Sometimes we're really crowded around the table, especially in the winter when we have extra staff and the students from the RN and aide programs are here."

The head nurse on the night shift flips through the Kardex (a file of cards with pertinent information on each patient) and updates each patient's progress for the day staff. Each nurse is usually assigned four to five patients for the day. Assignments are determined by the seriousness of the patient's condition and by the education and experience of the nurse.

When report is over, the head nurse begins dispensing the morning medications (staff nurses may also give medications, as needed, during their shifts). The staff nurses take vital signs on their patients, and at 8:00 a.m. the breakfast trays arrive. After breakfast, the nurses give baths and other personal care, start treatments, and take patients to other areas of the hospital as needed. Patients' lunches arrive at noon, and after lunch there is charting and catching up to do until 3:15 p.m. punching-out time.

At 11:00 a.m. on one hot September day (it is not unusual to see 120° temperatures in Brawley), a 64-year-old man is admitted to Room 223 on the medical wing. The room is a pleasant two-bed unit with a bathroom at one end. It is attractively decorated in green and white with green curtains at the window.

But it's still a hospital room, and the patient, Sam Howser, slumps forward in the wheelchair, his head on his chest and his hands gripping the seat canvas. His breathing is labored. Mr. Howser shakes his head back and forth and murmurs quietly. His wife, standing by his side, rubs her husband's back and explains to the nurse, "He's been fightin' comin' over here for quite a while."

Yolanda Smith, RN, wheels the patient closer to the bed and helps to transfer him from the wheelchair to the edge of the bed, where he again assumes the slumped-over position and grips the edge of the mattress with white knuckles. The wheelchair is pushed out of the room, and a heavy scale is wheeled in.

"Mr. Howser, I'm going to check you over and get you admitted to our floor. This is the first time you've been here, isn't it?"

Mr Howser shakes his head up and down but avoids eye contact. He holds his arm out to his wife. She moves to his side and slips her hand into his.

Nurse Smith holds an electronic thermometer unit in her hand. While she attaches the disposable sheath over the probe, she explains to her patient, "I'm going to take your temperature now. Would you open your mouth for me?"

Mr. Howser allows the nurse to put the thermometer under his tongue but almost immediately begins crying. Nurse Smith removes the thermometer, puts her arm around his thin, shaking shoulders, and asks, "Can you tell me what's the matter?"

"I don't want to stay here."

"I understand how you feel. But you're here to get better. The doctor wants you to have some special medicine for your breathing—you'll be getting it through this tube."

Nurse Smith puts down the thermometer unit and picks up the IV tubing that is attached to a hanging bottle at the head of the bed. "The fluid will go in your veins and there'll be medicine in it so you can breathe better."

"My veins aren't good."

Mr. Howser holds out his right arm and runs the fingers of his left hand up and down his right arm. He points to areas on his skin where blood has previously been drawn.

Ms. Smith speaks soothingly: "Our nurses here are very good at starting IVs."

Tina Pendley, RN, enters the room with tubes and other equipment for starting Mr. Howser's IV. "I'll do Mr. Howser's blood work at the same time I start the IV so I'll only have to stick him once."

Mrs. Howser walks to Nurse Pendley's side and whispers, "I don't know how much they told you—he has emphysema, heart trouble, and diabetes. I brought all his medicine here for you to see." She lines up various sized bottles on the bedside table. "This is his circulation pill and this is his water pill and this is—"

Nurse Smith has weighed Mr. Howser and helped him into his hospital "Johnny shirt." The electric bed is raised several feet and the head is raised to almost a ninety-degree angle. Mr. Howser coughs and spits up a large amount of mucus. The nurse hands him a small basin and a tissue. He drops his head back against the pillow and heaves a sigh of exhaustion.

Nurse Pendley moves to the patient's side and again explains the need for the IV. She wraps a rubber tourniquet around Mr. Howser's upper right arm. As she applies antiseptic to an area of the forearm, an aide pokes her head in the door.

"Mr. Swanson has to go down to nuclear medicine for a brain scan. The technician's here with the gurney."

"O.K., thanks." Nurse Pendley removes the tourniquet and explains,

"I'll be right back, Mr. Howser."

Mr. Swanson occupies the other bed in Room 223. He is 96 years old, and he was transferred to the hospital from the local nursing home for treatment of a possible stroke. For the past two hours, he's been out of bed in a wheelchair. The nurses now transfer Mr. Swanson from the wheelchair to the bed. The wheelchair is removed and the gurney is brought into the room and rolled alongside the hospital bed. Nurses Pendley and Smith stand at the bedside and the technician and aide stand at the side of the gurney. They use the short undersheet to lift and move the partially paralyzed patient to the gurney. Once covered and strapped on, Mr. Swanson is ready for the trip to the first floor.

While washing her hands, Nurse Pendley remarks, "Everything seems to happen at once."

She returns to Mr. Howser's side and again examines his arm. She applies the tourniquet, smears on the antiseptic, and inserts the needle. The vein collapses. Nurse Pendley removes the tourniquet and needle and applies pressure to the stick site with a sterile gauze pad.

"I'm sorry, Mr. Howser."

The patient responds in a monotone, "Don't be—can't be helped."

As an afterthought, Mr. Howser makes a suggestion: "In the lab, they usually stick me here." He points to an area on his left arm. Nurse Pendley moves her equipment to the left side of the bed. "So this is your lucky arm?" She goes through the same steps as before, but this time the stick is successful. The blood samples are taken and the IV is started. "Mr. Howser, you really helped me out."

For the first time, Mr. Howser smiles.

Nurse Smith continues examining and questioning the patient. "I'd like to listen to your chest—just take some good breaths for me—"

When she's finished, Nurse Smith will write up the admission notes on the patient's chart. In several hours, Mr. Howser's doctor will visit the patient and write further orders for his care and the nursing supervisor will make out a nursing care plan.

Supervisor Sally Lessicka sits in the nurse's station and tends to paper work. As a working supervisor, most of her time is spent with such head nurse activities as passing medications, making assignments, supervising staff nurses, and consulting with physicians. She is also responsible for administrative tasks such as attending hospital policy meetings. On call twenty-four hours a day, Ms. Lessicka responds to and tries to help solve the staff nurses' problems— "Usually an error is made or there's a conflict with a doctor. The nurse first needs reassurance that we all make mistakes or have problems from time to time and that she's not alone in her troubles.

"Nursing is a stressful occupation. We get pressure from patients,

patients' families, the physician, and the administrator. And we really have very little control over that. We can't snap back at patients or their families—we're here to help them. But the one relationship we have some control over here is our nursing staff. It starts with the nursing director—she's very supportive and will always back us up in any disagreement with doctors. And, on the floor, all the nurses try to pull together to get the job done. We work as a team—that's one reason why our staff turnover rate is so low. Patients can see this, too—we give good nursing care at Pioneer's."

Chapter 2

What Is a Nurse?

Chapter 1 showed the diversity of the modern nursing profession. Nurses today serve in a great variety of roles and settings, but they have a common history of ever-increasing specialization and professional status. Nursing today has its own unique body of knowledge, research, and theory that sets it apart from other professions, and nurses are functioning in new and unique roles in our rapidly changing health care system. This chapter looks first at the history of nursing and then examines its contemporary development by describing some of these new and exciting roles.

HISTORY

Nursing care began with the beginning of human life. Nursing, which means "to nurture or nourish," has traditionally been a woman's profession, and as such, the history of nursing parallels the history of women's role in society. To study the history of nursing one must look at the total history of humankind in order to understand how certain periods were more promising and others less promising for the profession.

For many centuries, medicine and nursing evolved separately and had little contact. In modern times, though, the technical aspects of nursing have become closely linked with medical progress and practice and nursing practice has therefore become more complex. The theoretical basis of nursing, with its emphasis on care of the whole person, remains separate from medicine, however.

The first nurse was probably a cave mother who tended her sick infant. Throughout ancient times, nursing was carried out by the female members of the household. It wasn't until the Christian era began that an organized group of nurses existed. Deaconesses called upon the sick in their homes, much like modern visiting nurses. These women were of high social standing and they served in order to atone for their own sins. As acts of charity, the deaconesses would bathe patients, dress their wounds, and prepare meals. But their main emphasis was on the spiritual aspects of healing, and this intertwining of physical and spiritual care is still important to many nurses today.

It was during the Roman-Christian time that the first hospitals appeared. The very first was built by Fabiola, a rich Roman matron, in 380 A.D. In this early Christian era, nursing took on a religious and maternal role rather than the medical-healer role. Nurses were seen as nurturing mothers and as aides to physicians. Today many people still

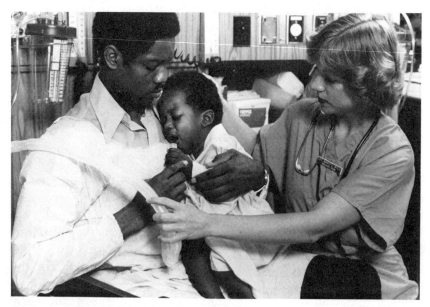

A pediatric nurse aids a father in giving respiratory therapy to his child. *(Courtesy Maternity Center Assocation)*

view nurses as adjuncts to physicians rather than as independent professionals, and many nurses find this view frustrating and difficult to counteract.

During the early middle ages, it was the nobleman's wife who cared for the sick in the feudal castle. As monasteries grew, the care of the sick became part of the community life of the monks. Nuns also provided medical and nursing care, and both Church and secular nursing orders sprang up throughout the middle ages. Nursing in the middle ages was very primitive and involved caring for the patient's needs as well as performing such tasks as scrubbing floors and carrying dirty linen to the river on wash day. During the time of the Crusades, men provided nursing care in military settings.

During the Renaissance (1500 to 1700), medicine began to emerge as a science. At the same time, nursing went into a dark period. The sixteenth century was the time of the Protestant Reformation, and Catholic nursing orders were repressed. Because of the new belief in individualism, care of the sick was no longer seen as a social responsibility. It was not until the late eighteenth century that the need for reform began to be felt. The eighteenth century saw the beginnings of our ideas about individual rights and social responsibility, and in particular our ideas about freedom for women, that led to the development of nursing as a profession.

In 1836 a hospital and training school for the deaconesses of Kaiserswerth was started in Germany. Kaiserswerth was a religious institution, but its primary emphasis was on rigorous educational preparation, not only in practical nursing techniques but also in pharmacy, anatomy, and physiology. It was the first truly modern school of nursing, and it was the school that Florence Nightingale attended.

Florence Nightingale

Florence Nightingale may be said to have created nursing as a profession, almost singlehandedly. Her remarkable organizing ability and strong personality enabled her to bring together in a practical way the social trends that underlay the foundation of nursing as a profession. These included rapid medical progress, which created the need for highly skilled nurses; improvements in hospital conditions; and the beginnings of women's emancipation. The training of nurses had begun to be organized in Protestant countries before Nightingale's time, but she placed nursing on a strong foundation of practical educational principles and created the first example of a profession administered by women. At the time of her birth, such an accomplishment was yet undreamed of.

Born in 1820 to a wealthy, socially prominent London family, Florence Nightingale was not interested in the usual feminine pastimes of her day. Receiving her education from her father, she preferred such subjects as math and Greek. Her experiences in caring for sick relatives convinced her that more than compassion was necessary for high-quality nursing—education was needed as well. At the age of 20, she pleaded with her parents to allow her to go to the Hospital Nursing School in London, but they refused. It's easy to see why. In England in the 1840s, hospitals were a place where the poor went to die, and nurses were of low character.

When her parents refused her, Florence sent away to European hospitals for information on training programs. During her European travels, she visited training institutions and social welfare organizations, absorbing all the information available about hospital reform and public health. Finally, at age 31, she stayed for three months at Kaiserswerth and participated in the deaconesses' training during that time. With her parents' blessing, Nightingale then obtained her first nursing position as superintendent of a small London hospital. She became known for her views on and knowledge about social welfare and was invited to become superintendent at a large London hospital, but her parents objected to her serving at a large public institution.

At this time, Russia was at war with the combined forces of England, France, and Turkey. Russia and France had religious orders to care for their armies but England had only untrained men to care for the sick and wounded. Cholera broke out and the wounded soldiers were placed in the filthy British hospitals of Turkey. The death rate was high. When Nightingale heard reports of these conditions, she decided she must go to help out. At the same time, the secretary of war (a long-time friend) urged her to consider going as a representative of the government.

Thirty-eight nurses went on this mission. They arrived at Scuturi in November 1854 and found conditions more horrible than they had imagined. The wards were crowded and many patients lay on the floors. Toilet and sanitary conditions were terrible, and equipment was nonexistent. In spite of this, the doctors did not want help from the nurses—they did not want women in a military hospital, and they resented the supposed slight to their abilities.

Nightingale began slowly. She opened five diet kitchens and started a laundry. As disaster fell on disaster at the hospital, the nurses were asked to do more and more. With her fine administrative skills, Nightingale brought order out of chaos, and she became a heroine both at the hospital and back home. As a special tribute, the secretary of war announced the formation of the Nightingale Fund to be used for the establishment of a nursing school.

In 1860, the Nightingale School for Nurses opened. It was the first fully endowed school, independent of any hospital. Nightingale felt that nursing was an art requiring organized, practical, and scientific training. She believed in a team relationship for the welfare of the patient and she felt that the sick *person* must be treated, not the *disease*. Insofar as doctors felt that nursing could be learned by intuition, Nightingale's one-year training school was a brave and revolutionary undertaking and had far-reaching importance for the establishment of nursing as a profession. What was this first school like?

Students awoke at 6:00 a.m. They worked in the wards from 7:00 to 9:30, making beds, giving baths, taking temperatures. At 10:00 they served "lunch." At 12:45 p.m., the students had their lunch and then helped with patients' dressings. At 2:00 there were lectures and a short rest, followed by tea at 5:00. From 6:00 to 8:30, the students fed the patients and got them ready for sleep. Back in the students' rooms, lecture notes were written up before lights went out. It was a full day.

After her military experience, Nightingale spent the rest of her life as an invalid. Although the nature of her illness is unknown, her role as an invalid enabled her to avoid social functions and unnecessary callers and thus have more time for her work. She directed her school and wrote volumes from her sick bed. Nightingale's popular *Notes on Nursing* was a practical, common-sense handbook on how to take care of the sick and also how to stay healthy. Much of its message is as worthwhile today as it was in 1859. In spite of her ill health, Nightingale lived until the age of 90.

Nursing in the United States

In the United States, the nursing profession has also closely followed the social, medical, and economic history of the country. In colonial America there was little organized medical care, and the few doctors who did practice were isolated from the scientific world of Europe. Women were nurses to their families and neighbors. If home remedies failed, a doctor was called. Only the very poor or homeless went to hospitals. As was true in Europe, the only good hospital nursing care was given by religious orders.

In the early 1800s, Dorothea Dix became a pioneer crusader for the mentally ill. For ten years, she worked to get a federal bill passed to give national aid to those who were mentally ill. She was appalled by patients who were chained, placed in cages, naked, beaten, and lashed. She traveled all over the country as an advocate for the mentally ill. As a result of her efforts, thirty psychiatric hospitals had been established before her death.

In 1861, during the Civil War, Dix was the superintendent of the U.S. Army nurses for the Union forces. Many religious orders volunteered to serve, and lay women were used to supplement the sisters. There was no Confederate army director of nursing. Hospitals were set up in tents, public buildings, trains, and steamers. Nursing care was given by volunteers.

Clara Barton, who served as a nurse during the Civil War, was instrumental in founding and organizing the American National Red Cross. Barton served as its head and later served as a nursing administrator during the Spanish-American War of 1898. The professional services performed by the nurses at this time changed many doctors' opinions of what nurses could do. In 1901, the Army Nurse Corps was established as a permanent organization, in 1908, the Navy Nurse Corps was authorized, and in 1949, the Air Force Nurse Corps was formed.

During the period between the Civil War and 1900 there was a great increase in the number and quality of hospitals in the United States. Health institutions have shown steady improvements and numerous reforms. Today, patients go to hospitals not to die but to receive the best care and treatment that medical and nursing science can offer.

As in England, war in America brought attention to the need for professional training schools for nurses, and the first such schools opened in the 1870s. By 1900, there were more than 500 schools of nursing and more than 10,000 graduate nurses.

In 1872, the New England Hospital in Boston admitted a class of five students to its newly formed one-year training school. Out of the five students, one person graduated. That was Linda Richards. For this student, there were no uniforms, no textbooks, no pre-entrance exams, no graduation ceremonies. After receiving a diploma, Richards decided on a position as night superintendent at Bellevue Hospital in New York. While there, Richards initiated the modern system of keeping written records and putting orders in writing.

Following this experience, Richards worked as superintendent of the Massachusetts General Hospital training school in Boston and then traveled to England to study English training methods and to meet

Florence Nightingale. She returned to the United States and started on a career of reorganizing the nursing services of hospitals throughout the country. In 1885 she went to Japan, where she organized and headed the first Japanese school of nursing.

During this period schools of nursing were rapidly established in the United States. All were modeled after the hospital apprentice-type program that had begun in England. Gradually, training programs increased in length, and coursework became more theoretical. New material was always being added to the curriculum. These changes were brought about through the efforts of dedicated nurse educators and administrators who were committed to the advancement of nursing as a profession. A few of the many milestones of these early years are listed here:

- In 1876, the first American nursing uniform was designed by a Bellevue student, Euphemia Van Rensselaer. It was a gray-blue striped floor-length dress worn with a white apron and cap. In the early years, the most conspicuous part of the apron was the utility bag that dangled from the belt. The first bags held a pencil, scissors, and a tiny case containing matches to light the candles and kerosene lamps. As the clinical thermometer and the hypodermic syringe were invented, these too were added to the bag (although stored in protective cases).

- In 1879, Mary Mahoney became the first Negro nurse to graduate from a school of nursing. Mahoney completed the sixteen-month program of the New England Hospital for Women and Children and went on to practice her profession for over 40 years. She was active in professional organizations for black nurses and worked to foster positive interracial attitudes among nurses.

- In 1893, Lillian Wald founded the Nurses Settlement, a neighborhood nursing service for the sick poor of the lower East Side of New York City. This was later to become the Henry Street Settlement. Wald was the first to use the phrase "public health nursing" and became the first president of the National Association for Public Health Nursing in 1912. She was active in promoting social welfare legislation, and it was due to her actions that the national Children's Bureau was formed. She was also one of the lecturers at the newly formed Department of Nursing Education, Teachers College, Columbia University. Wald was instrumental in getting nurses on the payroll at city schools and in organizing the Town and Country Nursing Service of the American Red Cross. Wald did much toward promoting the early and continuing relationship between nursing and public health.

- In 1895, a Vermont industrial company employed the first nurse to give care to sick employees. In this way, the specialty of industrial nursing began.

- In 1896, the Nurses Associated Alumnae of the United States and Canada was formed and became, in 1911, the American Nurses' Association. In 1900, the *American Journal of Nursing* was started; since 1912, it has been the official magazine of the American Nurses' Association.

- In 1898, the courses of Teachers College of Columbia University were opened to qualified nurses, and in 1899 a course in hospital economics was instituted. Thus nurses were for the first time considered to be qualified to work toward university undergraduate and graduate degrees.

- In 1903, North Carolina passed the first nurse registration act, and other states soon followed.

- As early as the turn of the century, it was suggested that education of nurses should be placed in educational institutions outside of the control of hospitals in order to make nursing more on a par with other professions. In 1909, the University of Minnesota School of Nursing, the first school of nursing integrated into a university, opened its doors.

- After World War I, the Rockefeller Foundation financed a study of nursing education. It was found that there were many weaknesses in the hospital apprenticeship program. In 1923, the Yale University School of Nursing was established with Annie Goodrich as its first dean. This school, which emphasizes advanced professional preparation, admitted and continues to admit only students who have already earned a baccalaureate degree.

- In 1952, the first technical nursing program, or two-year associate-degree program, as conceived by Mildred Montag, was opened in Middletown, New York.

- In 1952, the National League for Nursing (NLN) was formed from the combined resources and activities of three national nursing organizations, the National League of Nursing Education (founded in 1893), the National Organization for Public Health

Nursing (founded in 1912), and the Association of Collegiate Schools of Nursing (founded in 1933), and four national committees. The NLN is the accrediting body for all nursing education programs. Membership in NLN is open to nurses and non-nurses interested in improving health care education and practice. (More information on NLN and other nursing organizations appears in Chapter 5.)

- In 1953, the National Student Nurse Association was founded to improve conditions for student nurses and to serve as an information network.

- In 1972, the New York State legal definition of nursing established the professional status of nurses. For the first time in the history of nursing, it described the nurses' functions and established legal authority for the independent role of the nurse practitioner.

As nurses continue to move into areas that were once felt to be totally in the physician's domain, licensing laws (which control who enters the profession) and practice acts (which define the scope of the nurse's duties) will change. Nurses are held legally accountable for their actions: they are independent in their practice and interdependent with other health care practitioners, such as physicians. Further legal and legislative enactments will be important in determining the role of tomorrow's nurse.

Nurses today are the product of their past and change will be an inevitable part of nursing's future. In recent years, advanced practice in nursing has taken on a more specialized approach. Nursing is still mainly a woman's occupation, and as such it struggles to become independent and faces many of the same issues that all professional women face. As more men become nurses, they may have a profound effect on society's image of the nurse.

The professional lives of a wide variety of today's nurses are described in this book. These nurses are, day in and day out, making nursing what it is and what it will be. There are many challenges ahead and new frontiers need to be overcome. What will your place be in nursing's future?

DEFINITION OF NURSING

What is your image of a nurse?

In 1859, Florence Nightingale explained her vision of what nursing should be: "What nursing has to do is to put the patient in the best condition for nature to act upon him." One hundred years later, Virginia Henderson (a well-known nurse and educator) defined nursing as "assisting the individual, sick or well, in the performance of those activities contributing to health or its recovery (or to a peaceful death) that he would perform unaided if he had the necessary strength, will or knowledge. And to do this in such a way as to help him gain independence as rapidly as possible."[1]

Still another definition of nursing, developed by the American Nurses' Association, is, "Nursing is the diagnosis and treatment of human responses to actual or potential health problems."[2]

All three of these definitions tell what nurses do for their patients. But the work a nurse accomplishes depends on where she works (hospital, nursing home, health agency) and what area of health care she's in (an intensive-care nurse performs many complicated tasks to improve the patient's physical condition; a psychiatric nurse, on the other hand, gives psychological support and helps the patient to gain emotional health).

In Florence Nightingale's era, many of the nurse's tasks had to do with housekeeping, meal preparation, and patient hygiene. But by 1940, nurses performed almost all of the skills that had been the doctor's domain in Miss Nightingale's time. And today, many of the doctor's tasks of the '40s are now performed by nurses. Nurses not only change dressings and take blood pressure readings, they also do physical examinations, give injections, and handle sophisticated monitors and other machines. The list of what nurses do is almost endless and it's constantly changing.

But a nurse's role is more than tasks delegated by physicians. Nursing is a unique profession with a theoretical basis all its own. Nurses focus on the whole patient in sickness and in health.

Nurses are present at the most critical times in a person's life—at birth and death, at times of joy and sorrow. They are also present in the patient's everyday struggle of staying healthy and getting by. Nurses give care with all the scientific skills that are available to the twentieth-century practitioner. But they also touch patients, with their hands and their hearts, and this practice is as old as humankind.

---

[1]Virginia Henderson, "The Nature of Nursing," *American Journal of Nursing* 64:63, August 1964.
[2]This definition is based on language proposed in 1970 by the New York State Nurses' Association. This language was adopted as part of the Nurse Practice Act of New York State in 1972 and later incorporated in the nursing practice acts of several other states.

The art of nursing—keeping the human connection—that's what sets the nurse apart. That's her strength and her greatest contribution to society. Nursing is a difficult profession today when nurses are asked to do so much. But that, after all, is the essence of the nurse's world. To be a good nurse is to have compassion. A nurse must possess strong scientific knowledge and skills and also have that reaching-out quality of tender care and concern. Sounds like a lot to ask, doesn't it?

Titles

One of today's problems for the profession is the confusion over titles. Many times when you hear the word "nurse" you're not sure who is meant. It could be a registered nurse, a licensed practical nurse (LPN), a nurse practitioner, or any of the other designations that are often heard but frequently misunderstood.

To clear up some of the confusion, a few titles and explanations follow:

RN. RN stands for "registered nurse." A person who can put "RN" after his or her name has graduated from a school approved by the State Board of Nursing and has passed the State Board licensing examinations. Nurses may be licensed in more than one state, either by examination or endorsement of a license issued by another state. This license must be renewed periodically, and in some states, continuing education is required before an RN license may be renewed.

A candidate becomes eligible to take the State Board exam by graduating from a two-year associate degree program, a three-year diploma program, or a four-year baccalaureate program. Advanced degrees—MS and PhD—are also awarded in nursing. Educational preparation often determines salary and mobility within the field of nursing, and two levels of RNs may be said to exist in current practice—professional nurses, or those with baccalaureate degrees, and technical nurses, or those with associate degrees or nursing diplomas.[3]

Certain specialties in nursing require a minimum baccalaureate degree. (See Chapter 4 for descriptions of different programs of study.)

NURSE PRACTITIONER. Nurse practitioners have been called "super nurses" because of their high level of technical skills. A nurse practitioner (NP) is an RN with advanced training, usually as part of

---

[3]National League for Nursing, "Position Statement on Nursing Roles—Scope and Preparation" (New York: The League, 1982).

a master's program in nursing, who specializes in one area such as pediatrics, geriatrics, psychiatric-mental health, family practice, or midwifery.

The NP may be the first health professional that the patient sees and so provides basic primary care. The nurse practitioner performs many tasks that were once thought to be solely within the physician's domain. This includes history taking, physical assessment, patient education, screening and management of routine health problems, prescribing medications within the scope of the nurse's practice, counseling, and referral to other health care providers as needed.

Each state regulates NPs through the state's nurse practice act. In some states, NPs have been able to practice without significant changes in existing statutes. In states that prohibit nurses from engaging in diagnosis and prescribing treatment, NPs cannot practice without new statutory authority. The response of these states has been either to replace previous statutes with new definitions of nursing roles or to amend existing law to accommodate expanded-practice nursing. There is still considerable variation in the type of reimbursement that third-party payers offer for NP services. (For more on nurse practitioners, see Chapter 9.)

CLINICAL SPECIALISTS.   The clinical specialist's role differs from that of the nurse practitioner in philosophy and practice. Whereas the nurse practitioner works closely with doctors and in some cases makes medical decisions, the clinical specialist is the nursing expert or the practitioner of advanced nursing. A clinical specialist usually possesses at least a master's degree in her specialty area (this could be medical-surgical nursing, maternal-child health, mental health nursing, or another specialty area). A clinical specialist must also meet the eligibility requirements for certification.

Clinical specialists usually work in acute-care hospitals and give direct nursing care or advise other nurses on the care of those patients falling under their areas of specialty. The clinical specialist may also carry out nursing research and act as an advisor to various groups within the hospital. (For more on clinical specialists, see Chapter 8.)

PUBLIC HEALTH NURSE.   Also an RN, the public health nurse has a minimum baccalaureate education. Public health nurses work in the community and are usually connected with a health department. In the past, the title public health nurse was conferred after the nurse passed a civil service examination. Now the title is less clear and is often used interchangeably with that of the community health nurse.

Public health nurses visit homes and give some direct patient care and supervise other health workers in such care. In addition, they teach and counsel on an individual basis, assist in clinics, and speak to community groups. They work with physicians, hospitals, and other agencies to improve the health and well-being of the community. The emphasis of public health nurses' practice is the community as a whole; thus they have special skills in statistics, community assessment, and epidemiology.

VISITING NURSE.   A visiting nurse is an RN but not necessarily a public health nurse. The emphasis for the visiting nurse is on the individual patient rather than on the community at large. Visiting nurses may work for a nonprofit agency, such as a visiting nurse association (this is where the title originated), a private profit-making agency or a hospital-based agency. In all cases, they give direct care in the home.

In recent years, home health care has become more technical and complex so that many agencies require that their nurses have a minimum baccalaureate education. (For more on public health nurses and visiting nurses, see Chapter 7.)

LPN/LVN.   LPN/LVN stands for licensed practical nurse (in California and Texas, they are called licensed vocational nurses). An LPN is a graduate of a state-approved school of practical nursing and has passed the State Board examination for practical nursing. The length of the educational program varies but is usually one year at a vocational technical school or community college. An LPN works under the direction of a physician, a dentist, or an RN and provides routine technical care. Most LPNs work in hospitals, nursing homes, or doctors' offices and are responsible for delivering routine bedside care. The LPN does not have the educational background to provide the skilled care that an RN can provide, receives a lower salary, and does not have opportunities to move up within the nursing profession.

A person cannot become a licensed practical/vocational nurse by taking correspondence courses.

NURSING ASSISTANTS.   Also known as aides or orderlies, hospital attendants, auxiliary nursing workers, geriatric aides, psychiatric aides, or counselors and home health aides, assistants provide care to patients in institutions or in the home under the direction of a registered nurse. Training is usually short (six weeks to three months) and takes place on the job. There is no license or standardized examination for nursing assistants. In the community, nursing assistants are called home health aides. They work in the patient's home under the supervision of a nurse. In this setting, the aide may also plan and prepare meals, do food shopping, observe the patient's progress, and report findings to the supervisor.

In the broadest sense, every person who gives hands-on care or ministers to a sick person is a nurse. However, the term "nurse" is a legally protected title in many states, and when I use the term "nurse" in this book, I usually mean an RN and the specialties of her profession.

Read on, then, and see what your place is in this dynamic and necessary profession.

CHAPTER 3

Who Should Be a Nurse?

There's no other person with the same experiences, characteristics, interests, aptitudes, and abilities as you have. The more aware you are of the special qualities that make you *you*, the easier it will be to make a satisfactory career choice.

You probably have an interest in nursing or you wouldn't be reading this book. But is your interest based on experiences in the health care field or is it based on what you've seen on TV, in the movies, or in popular novels?

INTERESTS, APTITUDES, AND ABILITIES

So you have an interest in nursing. Do you also have an aptitude for nursing? An aptitude is not a skill or an ability but a talent that is undeveloped and untrained. It is a natural tendency to do well in certain areas. The best career choice is made when a person selects the field in which he or she has the aptitude, time, and money to follow through.

Because of the wide range of positions available in nursing, it's harder to pinpoint aptitudes for a nursing career than aptitudes for a career in, say, accounting. But there are some basic questions you can ask yourself:

1. Do you like math and science? Have you gotten good grades in basic math and science courses?

2. Do you work well in emergency situations? Do you have common sense?

3. Do you meet new people easily? Do your friends say you're a warm and friendly person? Do you prefer being around others rather than being alone?

4. Are you intrigued by machines and have an interest in how they work?

5. Do you find satisfaction in helping other people?

6. Do you work well with your hands?

7. Can you think problems through logically?

8. Can you express yourself effectively in speech and in writing?

9. Are you an independent, creative person?

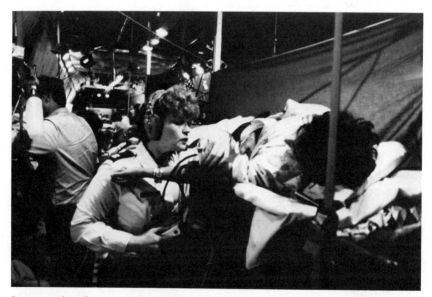

Do you work well in emergency situations? A U.S. Army nurse checks blood pressure. *(Courtesy U.S. Army)*

For the prospective nurse, all these questions deserve a yes answer. I'll explain why.

Nursing is part of the health science field. In nursing school, you will be required to take many science courses. On the job, you will use your scientific knowledge to give effective patient care. If, as a high school student, you've found biology, physics, and chemistry challenging and seldom boring, and if you seem to have a natural curiosity about the world of science, then nursing may be for you. If you get good grades in these areas, that's usually a good indicator of scientific aptitude.

Abilities in basic math and quantitative reasoning (solving word problems in math) are also important in nursing. Math skills are used on the job to calculate drug dosages and determine proper treatment. Most important, a nurse needs to think clearly and logically—a patient's life may depend on this ability.

The modern nurse has to learn how to use many sophisticated machines and other devices. In the educational setting, the student is taught these skills, and in the clinical setting, experience will prove an even more effective teacher. Modern technology, and the gadgetry that it entails, is very much a part of nursing today.

But nursing throughout history has been a helping profession. It still is. If you don't like working with people and relating to people and helping people, this profession is probably not for you. Also, nursing lends itself to the unusual rather than the usual. It is never dull or routine. So being creative, being able to "roll with the punches" and make independent decisions—these are all important qualities to have. In the beginning, of course, you won't feel too confident. No student nurse does. But if your basic personality is one of confidence and self-assurance, you should do well.

Effective communication skills are a requirement in nursing. Nurses teach patients and family members, delegate tasks to those who serve under them, and interact with doctors and other health care personnel. They write nursing plans and chart patients' progress. As a nurse moves up through the ranks and takes on more responsible positions, communication skills become even more important.

Lastly, nursing is hard work, hard both physically and emotionally. Nurses are required to be on their feet, moving about, and doing physically demanding tasks. It takes a person who is physically well and emotionally stable to pursue a career in nursing.

Do nurses have a morbid interest in sick people or do they "love" the sight of blood? No. Health professionals recognize that unpleasant sights and smells may accompany illness. Nurses do not enjoy the sights of illness, but in their desire to help others attain wellness they learn to cope, become accustomed to their special role, and focus their attention on the needs of their patients.

If I were to profile the perfect nurse (and, of course, there are few of those around), I would list the following qualities as most important for *all* nurses:

Nurturing—compassionate

Science aptitude—technical skills

Adaptable—creative

Able to communicate effectively

Physically fit—emotionally stable

Advantages of a Nursing Career

But why be a nurse at all? When there are so many other career opportunities, why consider nursing? There are many advantages to being a member of this valuable profession.

Serving Mankind. A nurse helps at the most important times in a person's life. Be it birth, death, serious injury, or disease, the patient needs help and is grateful for the care the nurse can give. The satisfaction of relieving a person's pain or fear and being able to see the results within a short time is a real bonus for nurses. A "thank you" is nice, but more important for the nurse is seeing a once very sick patient get better and leave the hospital to take up his or her life again. The satisfaction of knowing you were able to help—of knowing your skills and abilities made a difference—is the greatest reward in nursing.

Respect. Nurses are respected members of the health team and of society. Whether in the hospital, in the community, or in the nurse's own backyard, a nurse is considered a competent resource person who is held in high esteem.

Diversity of Employment. In Chapter 1, nurses in four different fields were highlighted. Their day-to-day work is vastly different, yet they all put "RN" after their names. There are a tremendous number of specialities within the profession and a nurse can select from a variety of positions in any part of the world. With additional education and training, it is relatively easy to change specialties within the profession. Besides the careers detailed in this book, there are many more that are being pursued by ambitious health professionals. Want to combine nursing and communications? There are positions for nurses in writing, public relations, and health education.

Uniqueness of Profession.　　"Nursing is the only discipline that looks after the patient's total health needs over a 24 hour period," says Carol Scales, RN, MSN, Director of Nursing at Whiting Forensic Institute in Middletown, Connecticut. "Nurses understand what's happening—with their patients and with other agencies. As a result of DRGs (see Chapter 6) and the new planning that's required, nurses are in a unique position to problem solve and act in the patient's best interests."

Scales continues, "Nurses have a great amount of freedom to be creative and the field is wide open for nurses with innovative ideas."

The profession of nursing has always been "people-oriented." Today's health consumer appears to be looking for just the kind of personalized, humanitarian care that nurses have always provided.

Personal Considerations.　　There are few careers that offer the time flexibility that nurses enjoy. Either part-time or full-time, hospital and nursing home nurses give care to patients around the clock, seven days a week, so nurses can work their own hours and still raise a family or continue their schooling.

To some practitioners, nursing is just a job that pays well enough to allow them to enjoy other areas of life. To others, nursing is a lifetime commitment with emphasis on professional growth and the hope of high-level positions. Both types of nurses will find comrades in the profession.

Nursing is a career that can be stopped and started up again as personal needs arise. Families move, children grow up, couples are divorced, husbands die—these are realities of life for many women. With a basic nursing preparation and brush-up education, a woman can find a secure, meaningful position in life and can become economically independent.

Nursing is an essential health care service. While other careers come and go, nurses—no matter where they practice—will be needed and will be able to find employment.

There are some other "reasons" for going into nursing that should be mentioned. If you're considering nursing because you value high salaries, then reconsider. Also, if you like wearing elegant clothes and being around glamorous, sophisticated people, nursing will not satisfy you. If you're looking for a low-key job, nursing is probably not for you either. Nursing, with its rich human experiences, is never dull. Quite the opposite—it can be very stressful and demanding. But the rewards often come when a nurse is able to solve the problems and meet the challenges that are part of the profession.

Sources of Information

To find out more about nursing, it's important to go to the right sources. You can begin now by talking with a nurse who's a friend of the family or a nurse you knew when you were ill. You can talk with your school nurse and perhaps help out in her office, or you can contact your local health care agency and spend some time with the community health nurse and see what her job entails. You can take the Red Cross first aid or home nursing course (*every* person should have proficiency in administering cardiopulmonary resuscitation, or CPR). Baby-sitting is a fine way to learn about growth and development of children. Girl and Boy Scout groups have badges that pertain to health and there are projects for helping certain groups, such as the handicapped or the aged.

Future nurse clubs are not as prevalent as they once were, but many high schools, colleges, and county medical auxiliary organizations sponsor career days for nurses. At one such conference, held at a large medical center hospital, a nursing educator spoke to the students about several specialties in acute-care nursing and then took the group on a tour of the hospital. At another conference, nurses from several types of work settings sat at a long table in a conference room and briefly described their specialties. A question-and-answer period followed the presentation.

In school, when you're required to write a paper and have a free choice of subjects, why not select some aspect of nursing and research this area to increase your knowledge? If you can participate in a science fair project, this is an ideal time to satisfy your curiosity and use the scientific method to find out the "why" of a topic that interests you. Substantial prizes are awarded for excellent science projects. Why not make yours health- or nursing-related?

At the end of this book, there's a list of reading materials that can help give an honest picture of the nursing profession, and in Chapter 4, I'll discuss actual prenursing jobs in various medical institutions, both paid and volunteer.

Another approach is to talk with a student nurse at a local school— you may even be able to spend the day with her. I visited several nursing schools and found that the students had a great amount of insight about the profession they chose.

TODAY'S NURSE

There are 1.5 million RNs in this country who are employed in nursing. But it's not enough. According to the American Hospital Association's division of nursing, the number of unfilled positions in hospitals in the United States has increased dramatically. In 1986, job openings for RNs more than doubled and the association expects that the situation may soon be desperate. Data from the hospital association indicates that the shortage is widespread and not limited to one area of the country or one or two clinical areas.

According to a study by the Institute of Medicine (IOM), nurses with graduate education are "a scarce natural resource." One estimate cited in an IOM study projected that the demand for nurses with master's degrees will reach 256,000 by 1990, while the actual supply is projected at less than half that number. The supply of doctorally prepared nurses is predicted to reach only 5,600 by 1990, in contrast to a projected demand for nearly 14,000.

In addition, the Health Resource and Services Administration (HRSA), in its 1984 Report to the President and to Congress, estimated a demand for at least 964,800 baccalaureate-prepared nurses by the year 2000, compared to an estimated supply of between 466,000 and 519,000.

In terms of numbers, nurses are a powerful force. Where do most nurses work?

From *The Registered Nurse Population* (U.S. Department of Health and Human Services), the November 1984 breakdown of full-time and part-time nurses was as follows:

Employment Setting	Percentage
Hospital	68.1
Nursing home/extended care facility	7.7
Nursing education	2.7
Community/public health	6.8
Student health service	2.9
Occupational health	1.5
Ambulatory care setting employee	6.6
Private duty	1.5
Other self-employed	.01
Other	.01

How much money do nurses make? Following are the average earnings for full-time registered nurses by various employment settings, as of 1984 (from *The Registered Nurse Population*). The average annual salary for all full-time RNs is estimated at $23,505. Breakdown by employment setting and position is as follows:

Setting and Position	Average Annual Salary
Hospital	
Administrative	$32,982
Supervisor	26,629
Instructor	25,931
Head nurse	25,931
Staff nurse	22,394
Nurse practitioner/midwife	27,970
Clinical nurse specialist	26,512
Nurse clinician	25,396
Certified nurse anesthetist	37,552
Researcher	24,858
Nursing Home	
Administrative	22,776
Supervisor	19,870
Head nurse	19,822
Staff nurse	18,220
Nursing education	
Administrative	34,576
Instructor	24,564
Community/public health	
Administrative	28,256
Consultant	23,929
Supervisor	23,181
Staff nurse	20,006
Nurse practitioner/midwife	22,689
Student health	
Staff nurse	19,310
Occupational health	
Supervisor	25,043
Staff nurse	22,969
Ambulatory care setting	
Administrative	29,259
Supervisor	21,035
Staff nurse	18,032
Nurse practitioner/midwife	27,655
Clinical nurse specialist	21,537
Nurse clinician	20,126

| Private duty | 21,585 |
| Other self-employed | 34,882 |

It should be remembered that these figures are estimated averages—salaries for individual nurses may be influenced by geographic area, individual employment setting, length of service, educational preparation, responsibilities, and other factors. For example, hospital nurses earn the most money in large institutions located in metropolitan areas. Hospitals run by the federal government traditionally pay the highest salaries. The higher a nurse climbs the career ladder, the more money he or she will make.

Nurses in specialty areas requiring additional education also earn more. Specifically, the average annual earnings of registered nurses by highest educational preparation is as follows:

Educational preparation	**Average annual salary**
Associate degree	$22,129
Diploma	22,963
Baccalaureate	23,995
Master's	28,763
Doctorate	35,743

Most hospital and nursing home nurses receive extra pay for working evening and night shifts and agency nurses make top hourly rates in all settings.

In terms of geographic distribution, *The Registered Nurse Population* found that average annual salaries ranged from low to high as follows:

East South Central	
New England	Low
South Atlantic	
West North Central	
Mountain	
Middle Atlantic	
East North Central	
West South Central	High
Pacific	

The average annual salaries in 1984 for this study of registered nurses in staff positions ranged from $19,914 to 25,018.

As was pointed out before, there is a shortage of nurses in this country. Most hospitals are actively recruiting for the vacant positions on their staffs and many are offering special incentives to prospective nurses. What accounts for this recent nursing shortage?

1.   **Our older population, increased medical technology, and changes in health services.** Because of improved medical care and other factors, people in this country are living longer. Older people have more health problems and require more services from the health care system than younger people. Because of DRGs, older people are staying in the hospital for a shorter period of time but they tend to be sicker and require more complex hospital care and also require continued nursing services after discharge. For this reason, the number of nursing homes and home health agencies has also increased and many nurses are needed to give care in these areas.

Because of advances in medical technology, more specialized treatment is being given to patients of all ages. It's only in recent years that patients have been given care in neonatal intensive care units, trauma units, intensive care units, cardiac care units, and burn units. The ratio of patient to nurse in these areas is often one to one around the clock.

Because of prepayment programs for hospitalization and medical services, adequate health care is now considered to be everyone's birthright. Health consumers are also more informed and demand a high level of care from the medical and nursing professions. As a result of these factors, there's more demand for nurses now than ever before. And the supply has not kept up with the demand.

2.   **Drop in nursing school enrollments.** Fewer students are graduating from high school each year as a result of the lowered birth rate of the 1970s. Students can be more selective in their career choices. Women no longer have to choose the traditional nursing, teaching, or secretarial work for their career. There are many other fields open to them, such as engineering, auto mechanics, or medicine. Because of a smaller student pool and increased options for women, statistics show there was a 13 percent drop in total nursing school enrollments between 1983 and 1985. Financial aid has also been cut back in the last eight years.

I believe that a baccalaureate degree in nursing is one of the best educational routes a man or woman can take. A student nurse learns life experiences and a practical skill as well as receiving a good general education. Once out of school, a baccalaureate nurse can always find a job (compare this with a BA in English or History), and, with a baccalaureate degree as a springboard, can jump off to many careers within the profession. A nurse is also a knowledgeable health consumer and a more effective parent.

3.   **Working conditions.** Overwork and stress are common in nursing. Long hours, inconvenient hours, and little rest have always

been a nurse's lot. But many nurses will no longer stand for these conditions. As the nursing shortage continues, too few nurses take on too large a burden, and career burnout is the result.

Also, nurses want to nurse. They don't want to do paperwork or housekeeping tasks or take abuse from doctors. As nurses become better educated and more assertive, they expect a greater amount of respect from physicians and administrators. And they want to have more say in working conditions and other aspects of their career. Generally, nurses are being heard and changes are being made.

Furthermore, nurses are in a unique position to change fields within the profession. Tired of hospital staff nursing? You can try private duty or branch out to community health nursing.

4.   Salary. Nurses do not receive compensation comparable to that of other college graduates. Over the years, nurses have taken on an increasing amount of responsibility and are held accountable for their actions. Salaries have not kept pace with this fact. Although, with the current nursing shortage salaries are on the rise and will be for a number of years.

Salaries for nurses have also not kept pace with those of other professionals with similar educational background and status (even those in other traditionally female occupations). As more women, nurses included, become primary wage earners in their families, salaries have become a very important factor in career choice and satisfaction.

An interesting fact is that nurses tend to increase their salaries more quickly by educational achievement than by clinical experience. This has a beneficial effect on the profession in that better educated nurses will stay in the profession (since they are more likely to be well compensated) and will have the expertise to make changes and upgrade working conditions.

CHAPTER 4

EDUCATION

WHAT PROGRAM OF STUDY?

Recent statistics compiled by the National League for Nursing indicate that there are 1,474 basic RN programs in the United States—459 offered baccalaureate degrees, 777 offered associate degrees, and 238 were diploma programs.

What are the numbers of graduates from the three basic RN programs? Again from NLN, this was the 1986 graduate breakdown:

Baccalaureate	25,107
Associate degree	41,212
Diploma	11,496
Total	77,815

It's often frustrating to a student considering a career in nursing to find so many different programs of study. There's the LPN/LVN program, and for RN preparation there are the associate degree, diploma, and baccalaureate programs. Why so many ways to be a nurse?

Looked at from a positive point of view, the diversity of education has been an advantage in getting a great many nurses with widely different talents and goals into the profession. And from the point of view of the health care system, nurses are needed at every level of preparation.

However, there is a consensus among nursing organizations in support of baccalaureate preparation for professional nursing practice. Both the National League for Nursing and the American Nurses' Association have endorsed a system of two levels of nursing practice, the professional level and the associate or technical level. The minimum preparation specified for entry into professional nursing practice by the NLN and ANA is a baccalaureate degree in nursing, and for entry into associate practice, an associate degree in nursing.

The trend toward education of nurses in institutions of higher learning is demonstrated by the following statistics. According to the U.S. Department of Health, Education and Welfare *'81 Source Book—Nursing Personnel,* an estimated 8.2 percent of RNs had achieved a baccalaureate or higher academic degree in 1952. In 1970, this figure had risen to 14.9 percent. Recent statistics from NLN indicate that 32 percent of 1986 RN graduates had attended baccalaureate programs. The most significant increase within this group was for RNs with diplomas or associate degrees returning for baccalaureate degrees. This number grew from 13,377 in 1974 to 41,112 in 1984. Also during this time period, enrollments in master's programs went from 7,924 to 18,822. Doctoral enrollments went from 482 to 1,696.

On a personal level, there are many factors that a student must consider when selecting a nursing program. Some of these are scholastic ability, career objectives, personal goals and philosophies, time, and money.

It is helpful to know what each type of nursing program offers. The next few pages provide descriptions of LPN, AD, diploma, baccalaureate, and master's programs. These descriptions are, of course, general, so prospective students should consult the catalogs and course descriptions of schools that interest them for more specific information.

PRACTICAL NURSING PROGRAMS

In the usual LPN/LVN program, the length of study is one to one and a half years. Although entrance requirements vary, most schools now require a high school diploma or its equivalent.

Advantages.   LPN programs require a relatively small investment in time and money. With this limited investment, a person can see if nursing is the right career choice. After passing licensing exams, an LPN can immediately work in a hospital. Since supervised bedside nursing is all that some workers want to do, becoming an LPN may be the best route to take.

Disadvantages. An LPN works in a more limited capacity than an RN and has little prospect of upward mobility in salary, responsibility, or status. If becoming an RN is your ultimate goal, it is more efficient, in terms of both time and money, to enroll in a program that offers RN preparation.

LPN/LVN programs offer training rather than general education programs. Most courses are taken in only one field—nursing—and students learn the "how to" rather than the "why" by doing tasks over and over again. LPNs are prepared to perform only certain tasks in certain settings.

There is increasing pressure on LPN/LVN programs to expand and upgrade their course content to prepare health workers who can work effectively in today's complex health care system. The result is that LPN/LVN programs are being lengthened and are beginning to resemble associate degree programs.

ASSOCIATE DEGREE PROGRAMS

In the associate degree program the length of study is two academic or two calendar years. Entrance requirements include high school graduation. Some programs require college preparation courses. In some community college systems there may be open admission policies and no tuition. In private junior colleges, high SAT scores may be required and tuition may be as high as $8,000 per year, with books, uniforms, fees, and room and board extra.

Advantages. Programs are shorter than baccalaureate programs and therefore save time and money. Schools are usually close to home, and this provides an additional economic advantage. Some programs are designed for part-time students. The average age of students in community and junior colleges is 30. Many men also attend AD programs, so the student population is often more diverse than in other types of programs. General education classes are taken with students majoring in other areas. On completion of the program, the student is prepared to take the RN licensure exam and receives an associate degree. Graduates, on entry into practice, are prepared to manage the care of a small group of patients with common, well-defined health problems, and to supervise ancillary workers, as well as to give bedside care to patients with common recurrent health problems.

Disadvantages. An AD program does not prepare nurses for leadership or administrative roles or for positions in community health nursing.

In a typical associate degree program, one-half of of the courses taken are in liberal arts, one-half in nursing. Nursing courses combine classroom theory with clinical practice in extended care facilities (nursing homes), hospitals, and community agencies. A sample curriculum is as follows:

First Year: First Semester

FRESHMAN ENGLISH I. Practice in expository writing and library skills. Reading and discussion center on the formal and informal essay.

PSYCHOLOGY OF PERSONAL DEVELOPMENT. An introductory psychology course emphasizing the maintenance of a healthy personality. Topics include dynamics of adjustment; the problems that an individual faces in adjusting to family, school, peers, and job; and the techniques of readjustment, such as counseling and psychotherapy.

HUMAN BIOLOGY I. Selected topics in microbiology, parasitology, pathology, physiology, and anatomy. Laboratory work includes microscope technique, dissection, embryology, and genetics.

NURSING FUNDAMENTALS I. Fundamentals of nursing principles and practices related to the basic physical, emotional, and social needs of the individual. Topics include nursing history, communication skills, mental health concepts, the nursing process, asepsis and hygienic care, nutrition, administration of therapeutic agents, and responsibilities of the nurse.

PHYSICAL EDUCATION.

Second Semester

FRESHMAN ENGLISH II. Types of literature—short stories, drama, poetry—serve as the basis for continued practice in writing expository themes. Research paper required.

HUMAN BIOLOGY II. Human anatomy, physiology, and pathology are discussed in lectures. Laboratory work includes microscopic study of tissues and dissection.

NURSING FUNDAMENTALS II.   The nursing process related to the individual's response to illness, injury, and stress. Topics include therapeutic communication, diet modification, infection control, restorative therapies and rehabilitation, and responsibilities of the nurse.

PHYSICAL EDUCATION.

Second Year: First Semester

ELECTIVE.

SOCIAL SCIENCE COURSE.

ELEMENTS OF CHEMISTRY AND PHYSICS.   A survey of the fundamental principles of physics and chemistry. Lecture and laboratory experiences deal with safety, measurement, mechanics, heat, electricity, atomic and molecular structure, gases, chemical equations, solving chemical problems, solutions, topics in organic chemistry, and biochemistry.

MATERNAL AND CHILD HEALTH NURSING.   The nursing process, related to the stages of family development and the child's adaptation on the wellness-illness continuum. Topics include growth and development, birthing, parenting, nurturing, and the responsibilities of the nurse.

Second Semester

ELECTIVE.

PHYSICAL AND MENTAL HEALTH NURSING.   The nursing process, focused on the individual with commonly recurring health problems. Topics include medical, surgical, and mental health dysfunctions, nursing strategies within the health care delivery system, and responsibilities of the nurse.

DIPLOMA PROGRAMS

The hospital diploma school is the oldest educational program for RNs. In the mid-nineteenth century, women were not admitted to most universities, and the skills and knowledge that were required of a nurse were quite limited. So, following the European example, nursing schools in this country began as hospital-apprenticeship programs.

The number of such programs has decreased from nearly 800 twenty years ago to slightly more than 200 today.

In the usual hospital diploma program, the length of study is three calendar or three academic years. Entrance requirements include high school graduation. Cost of tuition and other fees varies from $3000 to $5000 per year. In many schools, tuition is reduced with each year of education.

Advantages.   Patient contact begins early in the program and continues throughout the experience. Also, diploma programs are often less expensive than baccalaureate programs.

Disadvantages.   After passing the RN licensure exam, diploma graduates are readily employed in all beginning hospital staff positions, but they are not qualified for certain positions outside the hospital. If they return to school to obtain a baccalaureate degree, they must validate their prior nursing knowledge, since their nursing courses do not carry academic credit. They must also complete several general education and baccalaureate level nursing courses.

A typical curriculum for a diploma program is as follows:

First Year: Fall

HUMAN PHYSIOLOGY I.   Study of cellular structures, tissues, energy sources, the muscular system, the nervous system, and special senses.

INTRODUCTORY PSYCHOLOGY.   Scientific study of learned and innate behavior of humans and lower organisms; examination of some basic assumptions, concepts, issues, methods, and findings of contemporary psychology.

ENGLISH COMPOSITION.   The basic principles of writing applied to the 500-word essay: methods of development, patterns of organization, and standard composition formats. Sentence structure, usage, and mechanics.

INTRODUCTION TO GENERAL CHEMISTRY.   Fundamentals of general chemistry, including, but not limited to, atomic and molecular structure and their interactions.

PHYSICAL EDUCATION.

Winter

HUMAN PHYSIOLOGY II.   Study of the skeletal system, blood, circulation, respiration, the kidneys, and immunity.

INTRODUCTORY BIOCHEMISTRY. An introduction to the fundamentals of biochemistry, based in organic chemistry. Topics include description of biological compounds and their functional groups, the metabolic pathways involving these compounds, and the interrelationships between the pathways.

INTRODUCTORY SOCIOLOGY. Study of society, with emphasis on the elements of sociological analysis, social organization, culture, socialization, primary groups, social stratification, associations, population, ecology, and sociocultural evolution.

DEVELOPMENTAL PSYCHOLOGY: THE LIFESPAN. Methods of studying human development: critical analysis of theoretical perspectives of human development. Emphasis on development among various domains and developmental tasks related to each life stage.

Spring

HUMAN PHYSIOLOGY III. Study of digestion, metabolism, acid–base balance, the endocrine system, reproduction, and biorhythms.

NUTRITION. Basic principles of human nutrition, including application to personal health choices.

INTRODUCTION TO NURSING. Elements of nursing and the role of the nurse are discussed. The relationship of nursing to the health care system in the United States is explored. Components of nursing practice, including legal and ethical aspects, are identified.

MICROBIOLOGY. Fundamental concepts of microbiology, including classification, identification, culture, physiology, nutrition, and control of microorganisms, with emphasis on bacteria.

Second Year: Summer

INTRODUCTORY PHARMACOLOGY. Basic principles on which the study of drugs is based. Systematic study of selected major drug groups and appropriate drug therapy interventions.

NURSING CARE OF THE ADULT PATIENT IA. Beginning course in medical-surgical nursing: principles and concepts from the behavioral, physical, and social sciences are applied. The concept of holistic nursing care is integrated throughout the course, and the nursing process is used as a foundation for nursing practice. The concept of stress is introduced, and nursing care focuses on promoting adaptation to selected stressors.

SOCIOLOGY OF HEALTH CARE SYSTEMS.   A study of health care systems as major social institutions, and their social impact on societies. Cultural variations in the meaning of health and illness and the organization, personnel, and financing of various health care systems are explored.

Fall

NURSING CARE OF THE ADULT PATIENT IB.   This second medical-surgical nursing course continues to focus on the concept of stress and adaptation. Holistic nursing care is provided for selected adult patients; the application of the nursing process is expanded. Emphasis is placed on promoting adaptation to stressors affecting selected body functions.

ABNORMAL PSYCHOLOGY.   The nature of abnormal behavior: symptoms and dynamics of psychological disorders; theories and methods of therapy and prevention; understanding normal behavior through study of abnormal behavior.

Second Year: Winter

MATERNITY NURSING.   Holistic nursing care during the child-bearing and initial childrearing phases of life. Emphasis on childbirth as a family-centered event. Concepts relevant to selected high-risk mothers, infants, and families are included and applied. The basic principles of family planning and various gynecologic alterations of the adult female are studied.

MARRIAGE AND THE FAMILY.   Sociological, anthropological, and historical perspectives. The basic nature of the modern marriage and family; the changed function of the family in modern society.

GENERAL PATHOPHYSIOLOGY.   A survey of the common pathological conditions associated with each of the systems of the human body.

Spring

NURSING CARE OF THE ADULT PATIENT II.   This clinical nursing course focuses on the concepts and principles of rehabilitation and gerontological nursing. The effects of aging and physical disability on the individual, the family, and the community are studied. The impact of chronic illness and physical disability on health care in the United States is investigated, and long-range concerns of chronic illness and physical disability are explored.

PSYCHOLOGY OF LEARNING.   Introduction to theories, concepts, and experimental literature in learning. Special emphasis on classical, operant, and cognitive views of learning.

Third Year: Summer

PSYCHIATRIC NURSING.   The basic concepts and principles of psychiatric nursing: the use of developmental and interpersonal concepts of human behavior when intervening to promote mental health; the similarities of human relationships in psychiatric and nonpsychiatric settings; the application of mental health principles and psychiatric nursing techniques in a variety of psychiatric and nonpsychiatric settings; legal issues affecting psychiatric nursing; community efforts for the prevention of mental illness.

TRENDS IN NURSING HISTORY.   Historical trends that have affected nursing are presented as a basis for the study of the development of nursing and nursing education. An initial exploration of the privileges and responsibilities of the individual as a member of the profession.

ELECTIVE.   May include any of the following: Understanding Literature, Speech Communication, Group Dynamics, Statistics.

Fall

NURSING OF CHILDREN.   A holistic approach to the child and family. Interaction with children at various points along the health-illness continuum, with emphasis on the child and family undergoing stress and adaptation in physical, psychological, intellectual, spiritual, and social modes. Principles and concepts from the physical-biological and psychosocial sciences are employed to provide a rational basis for the nursing process.

INTRODUCTORY SOCIAL PSYCHOLOGY.   Study of the nature of human nature: development of personality in the group setting; thought in human beings; nature and development of attitudes and their role in individual behavior; and personality problems in modern society.

ELECTIVE.

Winter

NURSING CARE OF THE ADULT PATIENT III.   The effects of acute illness on the patient, the family, the health care worker, and the community; problems related to the total care of the acutely ill patient; principles of nursing in mass emergencies.

CURRENT TRENDS IN NURSING.   The responsibilities and opportunities of the nurse as a member of the nursing profession are studied. Current social, economic, and educational trends that affect the need of society for nursing care are considered.

ELECTIVE.

Spring

MANAGEMENT IN NURSING.   This introductory course in leadership and management focuses on the concept of stress and adaptation as applied to health care delivery systems, using the holistic approach to help the student explore the management and leadership factors that affect the practice of professional nursing.

BIOETHICS.   Consideration of issues of applied ethics as related to practices and developments in the biomedical fields.

ELECTIVE.

BACCALAUREATE PROGRAMS

The baccalaureate program combines nursing courses with general education in a four-year curriculum in a senior college or university. Students may be admitted to the nursing program as freshmen or after one or two years of general education or liberal arts courses. Entrance requirements for nursing students are similar to those for students majoring in other subject areas. Minimum SAT scores and high school GPA may be specified. Tuition costs (not including room and board) may vary from less than $500 per year for in-state residents at state-supported universities to $10,000 per year or more at some private schools (and at state-supported universities for non-residents). There are scholarships, loans, and work-study programs available to lessen financial strains.[1]

---

[1]See *Scholarships and Loans for Beginning Education in Nursing* (New York: National League for Nursing, 1987).

another day they're working on a medical-surgical unit, and on still another day, they're assigned to the intensive care unit.

For the hospital, an experienced float nurse is a real asset. She can fill in the gaps when patient census is high or when nurses call in sick. Since the successful float nurse is familiar with all areas of the hospital, she tends to be a flexible, self-confident, and versatile professional.

The ultimate in float nursing is the agency nurse or, to use the vernacular, the "pool" nurse. This nurse is hired by an agency, which is responsible for placing her in a hospital or home situation and is in theory responsible for the care she provides. The nurse can accept or reject an assignment. Some of the larger temporary agencies offer the usual fringe benefits to their employees, and nurses can select their own hours. The pay is usually as good as or better than that of permanent staff nurses.

For some nurses, working for an agency is the perfect solution to balancing obligations of family, career, and education. For others, it's confusing to be thrown into unfamiliar situations. The potential for error is much greater, and there is a question as to who is responsible when inadequate care is given. Many hospitals resent having to pay extra for nurses who are unfamiliar with their hospital routine, so they have their own pool of nurses that they can call on at short notice. They pay these nurses per diem (daily) wages. In most cases, this is a far better solution than hiring agency nurses, since the nurses are familiar with the employing hospital and the hospital knows the quality of care that the pool nurses can provide.

The agency or temporary nurse services should not be confused with registry services. A registry nurse is an independent contractor who gives private-duty care. She lists her name with either a professional or commercial organization, which acts as a broker in placing the nurse in a patient's home, hospital, or nursing home. The registry receives a registration fee or a percentage of the nurse's salary, but the nurse is hired and receives payment from the individual patient or family. The nurse also provides her own benefits (including malpractice insurance). The registry, in other words, acts only as a go-between for patient and nurse.

The following sections describe the work of hospital nurses in a variety of specialties.

HOSPITAL SPECIALTIES

Emergency Room Nursing

Tri-City Hospital, located in Oceanside, California, is a 348-bed public hospital. Because its emergency room serves three rapidly growing cities, it's one of the busiest in the county, serving almost 4,500 patients a month.

Tri-City is a base-station hospital, and calls are received in the emergency room (ER) from paramedics by mobile intensive care nurses (or MICNs). As on the TV show *St. Elsewhere*, patients are seen in the field by paramedics, who make initial evaluations and report to the MICNs by radio transmission. There are at least two nurses working every shift who are certified MICNs, and they handle all incoming calls. Using information received from the paramedic, the nurse evaluates the patient's condition and follows a certain protocol in prescribing treatment in the field and en route to the hospital. In this way, precious time is never wasted and the patient's outcome is much improved by early treatment. The ER physician is available at all times as back up.

Summer is the peak time in most emergency rooms, and the weekends are notoriously busy. On one Friday night in late August, there are on staff two emergency physicians and five nurses (one serves as triage nurse, two are certified MICNs). There's also one emergency technician, who assists the physician in surgically stitching wounds and applying casts, as well as one Spanish-speaking LVN,

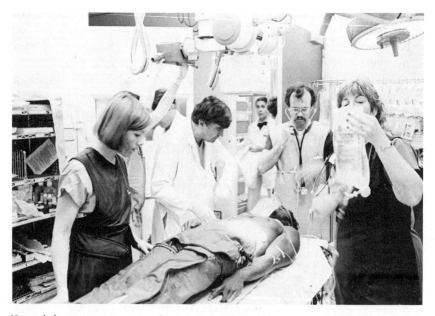

Nurses help to prepare a patient for an emergency X-ray.

who serves as interpreter when necessary. Two medical secretaries, several admitting clerks, and one volunteer complete the staff.

The triage nurse sees the patient first and sets priorities of treatment. Unlike appointments in a doctor's office, there is no "first come, first served" advantage. Patients are seen in the order of how urgent their problems are. A patient with a heart attack is seen before one with a broken leg.

At 7:30 p.m., a 5-year-old boy is brought to the emergency room by his parents. Around noon the boy had taken an overdose of his uncle's seizure medicine (a barbiturate, or "reds"). At 2:00 the boy fell asleep, and hours later the parents were unable to wake him. Placed in the treatment room equipped with monitors and other "crash cart" equipment, the child is immediately seen by the emergency-room physician, an RN (Joda Glassey), the LVN (who serves as interpreter for the Spanish-speaking parents), and members of the respiratory team. A medical secretary serves as scribe and records the observations and treatments made by doctor and nurse. To the casual observer, this would not appear to be an emergency situation—the team members speak quietly, work calmly, and coordinate their activities.

"B.P. 104/60" ... "respirations shallow" ... "pupils dilated but reactive" ... "responds to painful stimuli."

Lines are connected to the monitor, and Nurse Glassey makes sense out of the blips and bleeps: "Sinus tachycardia." A small mask is placed over the child's nose and mouth: "Oxygen on."

The doctor has ordered blood tests and X-rays. As each task is completed, the secretary records the time and the fact: "CBC done" ... "ABG done" ... Nurse Glassey calls out, "IV R/L (*Ringer's Lactate*) started left hand."

The LVN assists Nurse Glassey in inserting a tube through the child's nose and into the stomach: "NG tube down." They make sure that the tube is in the stomach, then irrigate, or *lavage*, the stomach with normal saline (a sterile salt-water solution): "Clear return." The youngster is restless and thrashes about on the narrow table. To keep the various tubes in place, Nurse Glassey applies restraints to the child's hands. Once these tasks are completed, Glassey gives instructions to another nurse, who takes over the child's care.

There's a loud buzz in the emergency area, and Joda Glassey quietly announces, "I'll get it." She moves quickly to the radio room and snaps on the button: "Tri-City Hospital." She listens to the paramedic; again there's the choppy medical vernacular: "57-year-old man" ... "short of breath" ... "past history emphysema" ... "respirations 42 with pro-longed expiratory phase." A specific medical protocol is followed in reporting and prescribing treatment. With a final message from the paramedic—"will transport ... ETA 10 minutes"—both parties give call letters followed by "Clear." Nurse Glassey completes the necessary paperwork and removes the tape cartridge from the machine. She explains, "All the tapes are reviewed by the coordinator, and once a week we have a base-station meeting. We can ask to have a particular tape reviewed at that time. We often do that if it's been a 'save' or a particularly difficult case where we did well. We like compliments the same as anyone else."

With the completion of this radio call, Joda Glassey finishes her ten-hour shift, although it will be another thirty minutes before she actually leaves the floor. Glassey will finish charting and report to the nurse who will be working the next shift.

Glassey explains the work schedule for ER nurses: "We work more flexible hours in order to provide the best coverage at the busiest times of the day. Nurses are offered the option of an eight-hour, ten-hour or twelve-hour shift."

The evening wears on and patients are brought into treatment cubicles. They are seen by nurses and doctors, receive tests and treatments, and are either admitted to the hospital or sent home. A 94-year-old women lies on a stretcher, propped up with pillows. Her diagnosis—congestive heart failure. Her family sits with her. There's a young man with a crushed foot—earlier that afternoon, he dropped a car transmission on it. There are patients with lacerations and broken bones; there's a boy who can't swallow a large lump of hard candy. A small child has an ear infection, and since it's now night and all the drugstores are closed, enough medicine is dispensed to last the night.

Nurse Sande Hoffman explains the typical work of an emergency nurse: "No course in nursing school really prepares you for work in the emergency room. The tasks are so varied and the pace is often very intense. You learn many of your skills on the job—that's why most of our nurses have been working in the emergency room a long time. It's hard to break in here—you have to be strong and independent. That's not always true in other hospital units. The doctors respect our opinions and we all work together as a team. Nurses frequently make suggestions to doctors on patient care."

Educational background of the nurses? "It varies from AD to baccalaureate nurses—the head nurse has an MS degree. Many of the day nurses have worked on the unit for ten years or more—they're very good. Many of them are three-year diploma graduates."

Besides the continuing education that is required of all California nurses, MICNs attend special classes and must continually upgrade their skills. It's very demanding, but a nurse receives extra compensation for being an MICN.

The loud buzz sounds and another MICN moves toward the radio room: "Tri-City Hospital." Within half an hour, two more patients are brought in by paramedics.

There's a toddler who's fallen from a swing set. She stopped breathing for a short time and was given mouth-to-mouth resuscitation by her mother. It's a potentially serious situation, so all staff members are alerted. The 5-year-old overdose victim is admitted to the pediatrics ward, and the large treatment room is prepared for the child who fell from the swing set. Within minutes, the child arrives on a wooden board—her head is braced with sandbags. An IV has been started in her right foot. The child is crying and talking and does not appear to be in any extreme danger. When she arrives, her mother is allowed in the room to comfort her while the physician examines the child. Skull X-rays and a CAT scan (a special X-ray) are ordered. Later she will be examined by a pediatrician.

Across the hall, the paramedics have brought in an 83-year-old woman who lives alone and fell in her bathroom at 3:00 that afternoon. She bumped her head and for a time was unconscious. Paramedics were called when the woman developed a headache and began vomiting. The nurse caring for her takes a history from the paramedics and questions the patient, who is now conscious. The woman is propped up on the stretcher, vital signs are taken, and the nurse starts the IV. The patient's level of consciousness is determined: "What year is this?" ... "What month?" ... "What city are you in?" The woman's answers are appropriate. The nurse explains, "She's alert now but I've seen patients with similar injuries who change quickly. Observation is very important in these first hours following injury." The doctor orders a CAT scan to check if there's bleeding into the brain as a result of the fall. The patient's private physician is called.

One of the nurses explains her feelings about working in the emergency room: "A lot of us complain about the work here, but probably none of us would want to be transferred. And there's this about the ER—maybe nobody else will say it—you don't get to know the patients as well here or at least not for as long as you do on the floors. That way you don't get as emotionally involved and you aren't as apt to get hurt. For me, that's a real advantage."

The pace seldom lets up, and as midnight approaches, the type of medical problems change. Sande Hoffman explains, "This will start the alcoholic and overdose cases and the gunshot wounds—after all, it's Friday night." The emergency physician, sitting nearby, comments on his co-workers: "A nurse here has to be really sharp and definitely has to have a coping personality. And this is one place where a nurse must be assertive. In emergency room work, a nurse either loves it and stays or hates it and leaves. There's nothing in between."

Medical Nursing

Every hospital has an emergency room and many patients are admitted to the hospital through this route. Patients seen in emergency rooms are suffering from acute illnesses or acute flareups of chronic illnesses. An explanation may be in order:

Acute illnesses, such as colds, pneumonia, broken bones, serious wounds, and food and chemical poisonings, produce signs and symptoms soon after exposure to the cause. An acute illness lasts a short time and there is either full recovery or the patient dies suddenly.

A *chronic illness*, on the other hand, produces signs and symptoms within a variable time after exposure to the cause. Chronic illnesses last a long time and go through periods of remission (when symptoms subside) and exacerbation (when symptoms recur). Some examples of chronic illnesses are asthma, emphysema, arteriosclerosis, arthritis, cancer, diabetes mellitus, hypertension (high blood pressure), and heart disease.

A patient with a serious acute illness is usually admitted to a critical-care area within the hospital (critical-care nursing will be discussed later in this chapter). Some patients with acute flareups of chronic illnesses are also admitted to these units, or they may be admitted to the medical floor. Certainly when the condition of a patient of either type stabilizes, the patient is transferred to a medical unit.

A medical patient is an adult who is receiving *diagnostic, therapeutic,* or *supportive* care that is not surgical or related to psychiatric therapy or the maternity cycle. A patient with a diagnosis of diabetes mellitus, for example, could be admitted to a medical floor for diagnostic tests (an angiogram, or X-ray of the blood vessels, would show the effects of atherosclerosis, a frequent complication of diabetes). Therapeutically, the patient might be placed on a strict diet and might receive a variety of medications, including insulin, to relieve the symptoms of this disease. The diabetic might receive support and teaching from the nursing and dietary staff on life-style changes, cause and course of the disease, insulin administration, urine testing, foot care, and so on.

Depending on the size and type of hospital, medical patients with different diagnoses might be mixed in together or there might be separate units for patients requiring services in the following areas of specialty:

1. Pulmonary disease (conditions affecting the lungs).

2. Gastroenterology (conditions of the stomach and intestines).

3. Nephrology (diseases of the kidney).

4. Cardiology (heart problems).

5. Endocrinology (metabolic disorders).

6. Orthopedics (diseases of the bones and supporting structures).

7. Neurology (diseases of the nervous system).

8. Gynecology (diseases of the female reproductive system).

9. Genitourinary (diseases of the male reproductive and urinary system).

10. Dermatology (diseases of the skin).

11. Hematology (blood disorders).

12. Rheumatology (arthritis).

13. Oncology (cancer).

14. Opthalmology (diseases of the eye).

15. Otorhinolaryngology (disorders of the ear, nose, and throat).

A staff nurse working on a medical floor has to be a generalist. All the clinical knowledge and skills learned in school—from chemistry to pharmacology, from psychology to rehabilitation—come into play. Adult patients are apt to be psychologically, as well as physically, out of sorts (a frequent word is "demanding"), and are at a very vulnerable period in their lives. Being hospitalized is a strain both to them and to their families. Nurse Lessicka, the medical nurse in Chapter 1, feels that "medical patients appreciate good nursing care."

The work that a medical staff nurse does tends to be more routine than that of a critical-care nurse, for whom one crisis follows another. On a medical unit, patients usually stay awhile and get to know their nurses. Patients with chronic illnesses are often hospitalized more than once. For the medical nurse, then, there is the opportunity to establish longer relationships with patients and families. This has both positive and negative implications.

Judith Gross, RN, is an assistant head nurse on a medical-surgical unit in a community hospital in St. Paul, Minnesota. She explains, "A nurse in this field must be practical by nature. She needs to be quick mentally and physically and needs to like people and have a good feeling for their emotional needs. She must be very adaptable, able to change course in midstream and not lose sight of previous objectives."

In her position as assistant head nurse, Nurse Gross is continually in touch with patients, doctors, nursing management, and workers in various hospital departments. It is her job to make sure that the unit runs smoothly, so she works closely with the nursing staff, serving as both role model and leader. She concludes, "The best part of every nurse's job is when a patient says, 'You've really helped me.' That means a lot."

Many nurses specialize in certain medical problems and have extra responsibilities. An orthopedic nurse, for example, has to work with traction equipment and other complicated devices. As one nurse stated, "To be a good orthopedic nurse, it helps to have a strong background in physics and a strong back!"

Nurses who deal exclusively with cancer patients and those who work with patients receiving kidney dialysis are some of the new nursing specialists discussed later in this chapter.

Surgical Nursing

Some smaller hospitals combine patients with medical problems with patients undergoing surgery on the same floor or ward. Larger hospitals do not.

Surgery is considered to be either *elective* (the trip to the hospital is planned and is at the patient's and doctor's convenience) or *emergency* (the surgery is performed as a life-saving measure and is done on short notice). Orthopedic surgery for hip replacement is an example of elective surgery, whereas an appendectomy is emergency surgery. Another way to classify surgery is whether it's done to cure or diagnose a condition, to alleviate symptoms (without curing the disease), or to reconstruct some body part to more normal appearance or function.

Whatever the reason for surgery, the hospital and nursing care is very similar. Jody Carlson, a surgical nurse who works at a health maintenance organization (HMO) hospital in Southern California, explains her work: "Much of what we do here is routine. We admit patients, see that papers are signed and that blood work and other tests are done. The surgical area is shaved and scrubbed the day before surgery, and patients are not allowed to eat or drink after midnight. Operations are usually scheduled in the morning and there is a certain

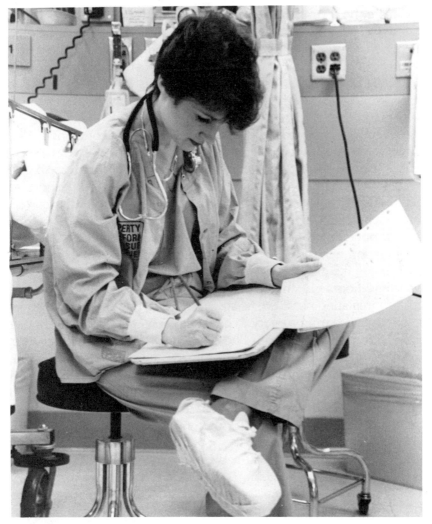

An O.R. nurse prepares her charts. *(Photo by Mary Belich)*

time for giving medications and doing certain tasks. But even though it's routine, it's different for each patient. Some need a lot of emotional support, or sometimes it's family members that need a caring person. Because the nurse spends the most time with the patient in those critical hours before surgery, she is the one who sets the tone and can make the difference in a patient's recovery."

Once the patient is transferred from the hospital bed to the gurney and wheeled to the operating suite, the responsibility for care lies with the surgical team. The doctor and assistants, the anesthesiologist or nurse anesthetist, the scrub nurse or technician, and the circulating nurse are the team members.

On TV, surgery is always carried out in an atmosphere of high drama. It is true that surgery is serious business (ask anyone who's been through it), and there's always the chance for bleeding or breathing emergencies or other complications. But most surgery is done within an established procedure. The procedure goes something like this:

The circulating nurse, an RN, assesses the patient's condition before surgery and talks to the patient, who is usually groggy from medication. The nurse's function is to help the patient, to reduce fear, to give needed information, and to provide emotional support. She also makes sure that the paperwork is in order and that all the correct instruments are ready. She transfers the patient from the gurney to the narrow operating room table and positions him according to the type of operation being done. The temperature in the operating room is cool, the lights are bright, and the machinery is polished steel. The walls and floors glisten, the air smells of antiseptic.

The circulating nurse wears surgical greens but does not scrub in, so she is free during surgery to get equipment, medicines, and other supplies for the surgical team. She keeps the records for the procedure.

The scrub nurse, who may may be an RN but is usually a technician, is the person who stands by the surgeon and slaps instruments into his hand. She also may hold the retractors to keep the wound open and cut sutures. But before she does this, she and the patient, as well as the surgeons, must get ready for the operation.

Strict asepsis is practiced in the operating room and all instruments and equipment are sterilized (made free from live organisms). Before every operation, the surgeon, assistants, and the scrub nurse scrub their hands and forearms with a sterile brush and antiseptic detergent for a prescribed period of time. After scrubbing, the hands and forearms are blotted dry with a sterile towel, and the surgeon and scrub nurse put on sterile gowns and gloves. They also wear masks, caps, and covers for their shoes. All these measures are taken to prevent spread of disease-causing organisms.

After the patient is anesthetized, the surgical site is again thoroughly cleansed. The surgical field is then draped with sterile towels and there is a wide sterile area around the operative site. It is only when all is ready that the surgeon begins the operation.

Operating room nurses are on their feet a great deal and much of the work that they do is repetitive. A knowledge of anatomy and physiology is essential for all OR personnel, and they must know the routine and procedure of individual surgeons. A scrub nurse (or technician) must be quick with instruments and should be able to anticipate what is needed without being asked. Although much that occurs in the OR is routine, changes can occur rapidly, and nurses may be called on to use quick judgment.

Following surgery, patients are transferred either to the recovery room or the intensive care unit. The recovery room is the more usual place, and the patient stays there until out of danger. The recovery room nurse observes the patient carefully for bleeding and after effects of anesthesia. She monitors the vital signs frequently and gives pain medication as needed.

When the vital signs are stable (or, in the case of spinal anesthesia, when feeling has returned to the legs), the patient is returned to the surgical floor. Surgical nurses in the post-op area are not known for pampering patients. They get surgical patients out of bed early and insist that, while in bed, they "turn, cough, and deep breathe" to prevent lung complications. Surgical nurses on this unit must have keen observation skills and must understand what each operation involves and what the common complications are. In times of emergency, surgical nurses must be able to act decisively. Depending on the type of operation performed, patients usually experience a gradual recovery and leave the hospital for a final recuperative period at home.

Nurse Anesthetist

Jeanne Hoffman is scheduled for a hysterectomy (surgical removal of the uterus) and checks into her local hospital the afternoon before the day of surgery.

After getting settled in her room, one of Hoffman's first "visitors" is Christine Zambricki, certified registered nurse anesthetist (CRNA). Zambricki reviews Hoffman's chart, then takes a health history and examines her patient, paying particular attention to any problems in the chest or airway that may interfere with anesthesia. This is also the time when Zambricki discusses the various types of anesthesia and determines which one will be most appropriate. Mrs. Hoffman is quick to voice her concern, "I've heard this can be a painful operation. Is that true?"

"If you have pain following the surgery, we have medication that can help you. And we'll give it to you as quickly as we can. There are some other strategies that can help in coping with the pain ... "

Zambricki describes some relaxation techniques. She also answers Hoffman's questions about what to expect after surgery, what special equipment may be necessary and what Hoffman will need to do herself to speed recovery and to prevent complications.

Following this initial visit, Zambricki contacts the physician who will be performing the surgery and discusses the type of anesthesia, anticipated length of surgery and other factors.

The next morning Jeanne Hoffman is prepared for surgery by the staff nurses. As Hoffman is wheeled to the operating room, Zambricki is finishing up morning conference with the anesthesiologist, other nurse anesthetists and graduate students. "This is a stimulating time when patient care plans are discussed (and challenged)," says Zambricki. "It helps us to get ready for the day's schedule."

By 8 a.m., Jeanne Hoffman has arrived in the holding area and Christine Zambricki, dressed in O.R. clothes, again reviews Hoffman's chart, then chats with the middle-aged woman.

"Do you remember yesterday we talked about the type of anesthesia you'd be receiving? I'll be putting a mask over your face as the anesthetic begins. When you wake up, it'll be over and it'll seem like only a few minutes passed. You'll feel very rested."

"Will you be with me when I wake up?"

"Yes, I'll stay until you're awake."

While they're talking, Zambricki has started an IV in Hoffman's arm, has wrapped the blood pressure cuff around the other arm and has attached the leads for the electrocardiogram (EKG). She will attach other monitoring devices once the anesthetic is in progress.

Hoffman is wheeled into the operating room and placed on the table. Zambricki explains, "I'm going to take your blood pressure now."

The anesthetist then positions herself near Hoffman's head and speaks soothingly to her patient, "You'll be going to sleep soon. Just relax and breathe normally."

Zambricki places a mask over Hoffman's nose and mouth and gives the anesthetic. Shortly afterwards, Zambricki passes an endotracheal tube into the patient's breathing passage and applies positive pressure ventilation. The surgery begins.

As Zambricki follows the necessary procedures and monitors her patient's vital signs, she notices that Hoffman's blood pressure has dropped slightly. Zambricki gives some medicine through the IV and adjusts the fluid but Hoffman's blood pressure is still at a low range. She alerts the surgeon, "B/P 100/60."

The surgeon removes some packing material, discovers a couple of "bleeders" (blood vessels that have not been closed properly and are oozing blood) and ties them off with sutures. Within ten minutes, Hoffman's pressure is back up to 120/80. To double check, Zambricki draws a blood sample and sends it to the laboratory. The hemoglobin test comes back normal which indicates the bleeding problem is under control.

As the surgical procedure continues, Zambricki monitors her patient's vital signs and adjusts the flow of the anesthetic agent as necessary. She continues to keep the surgeon informed about Hoffman's condition.

When surgery is completed, the anesthesia is discontinued and Zambricki accompanies Hoffman to the recovery room. Within a short time, Hoffman is awake.

"Is it over?"

"The operation is over and everything is fine."

Hoffman offers a weak smile then closes her eyes. After checking Hoffman's blood pressure another time, Zambricki leaves the care of her patient to the recovery room nurse although she will stop by and see Hoffman at least one more time during the recovery period.

Zambricki often takes time to find the patient's family and tell them that the operation is over and that the anesthesia went well. This is especially important when the patient is a child. "Sometimes family members get nervous," explains the nurse anesthetist. "They may have been told by the surgeon that the procedure would only last 15 minutes but they've had to wait for almost two hours. The other activities—such as preparing the patient—are what take up time."

After completing her care for Jeanne Hoffman, Ms. Zambricki returns to the holding area and prepares for her next patient. When all the surgical cases are finished for the day, Zambricki goes on rounds and visits patients who are scheduled for surgery the next day and also visits post-surgical patients to monitor their progress and make sure that quality care was given.

The nurse anesthetist carries a beeper with her and may be called at any time during the day to trouble shoot for airway management problems. In addition, she is a member of the cardiac resuscitation team that responds immediately to any cardiac emergency in the hospital.

The position of nurse anesthetist carries a great amount of responsibility and can be stressful. "There's not a lot of time between events if things aren't going well," says Zambricki. "However, a survey was published in our professional journal which stated that 80 to 90 percent of nurse anesthetists are satisfied with their jobs."

Today, more than 50 percent of an estimated 20 million anesthetics given in the United States each year are administered by nurse anesthetists. What exactly does it take to become a member of this specialty?

A nurse anesthetist is an RN who has specialized in the administration of anesthesia (physicians may also specialize in anesthesia—their title is anesthesiologist). If a nurse anesthetist's qualifications for entry into practice (including the successful completion of a certification examination) have been approved by the Council on Certification of Nurse Anesthetists, the individual may use the initials CRNA (certified registered nurse anesthetist) after his or her name.

According to the American Association of Nurse Anesthetists, in mid-1987 there were 20,980 active practicing nurse anesthetists (in 1971 there were 14,661). About 47 percent of all CRNAs are employed by hospitals, 38 percent by physicians, while 12 percent contract their services independently. In addition to working in the operating room, CRNAs may practice in psychiatric wards, emergency rooms or intensive care areas. Nurse anesthetists may also be employed by dentists, dental specialists, podiatrists, plastic surgeons and by the increasingly common ambulatory surgical centers, health maintenance organizations (HMOs), preferred provider organizations (PPOs), and other alternative care facilities.

To enter an accredited program of nurse anesthesia, the student must possess a BSN or other appropriate baccalaureate degree, hold an RN license, and have a minimum of one year's experience in an acute care area. The nurse anesthesia program ranges from 24 to 36 months, depending upon the type of degree offered. Students are given the opportunity to integrate classroom content with direct application of state-of-the-art techniques in providing anesthesia care to patients in all risk categories. Part of their education also includes experiences in the management of respiratory care and emergency resuscitative responsibilities in intensive care units, recovery rooms and other acute patient care areas.

There are 102 accredited nurse anesthesia programs in the United States. Many of these programs offer a Master's degree in such areas as nursing, allied health, and biological and clinical sciences. Other programs offer a course of study culminating in a professional certificate or baccalaureate degree. Once a student has completed his or her educational work, the nurse is eligible to take a national certification examination. The examination is given twice a year in testing centers throughout the country.

Christine Zambricki has been a certified nurse anesthetist for ten years. Her present position is administrative director of nurse anesthesiology at Mt. Carmel Mercy Hospital in Detroit. In addition, she is the program director of the graduate nurse anesthesiology program at Detroit's Mercy College. "In spite of my work demands—which often are administrative—I try to spend one day a week as a CRNA interacting with patients and being in the operating room. I like and need this contact."

Zambricki received her BSN from Michigan State University and her MS in nurse anesthesia from Wayne State University. After graduating, she worked as a staff anesthetist and was on the faculty at Wayne State University. Zambricki believes that the education of nurse anesthetists is unique in that most of the nursing skills are learned in the program rather than on the job. "Educational programs require that students have experience with at least 450 patients. Our students here care for 600 to 700 patients. Of course, learning never stops for the CRNA. New anesthetic agents and new techniques are constantly being introduced. Continuing education is very important and is mandatory (a minimum of 40 contact hours of approved CE programs are required every two years)."

Salaries for CRNAs exceed those of other nurses with the same educational background. The specialty also enjoys an amount of prestige not usually found in other specialties. Zambricki offers some advice, "I would suggest that if an RN is interested in being a CRNA, he or she should have an even-keeled personality and be able to stay in control when things are moving fast. In addition, the nurse should have good clinical judgment and be able to synthesize information and put it together in a new way.

"One very important quality is being assertive and being able to act as a patient advocate. The environment of the operating room can be difficult and the CRNA must be prepared to argue for the patient and quality care. The pay-off comes—for me anyway—in the intense relationship I enjoy with patients and knowing I was able to make a difference in their care and recovery."

Obstetrical Nursing

"Obstetrics is usually a happy service and it's a place where teaching by the nurse is well received, since new parents are very motivated to learn. Doctors on this service generally listen and respect the nurse's judgment, too."

At the 100-bed private San Diego hospital where Nurse Kay Yaussy works, the obstetrics service is located on one floor but is divided into three sections: labor and delivery, the sixteen-bed postpartum unit, and the nursery. Patients are admitted to a labor room and are moved to the delivery room for the baby's birth. They spend a short time in the recovery room, and then the babies are moved to the nursery and the mothers to the postpartum unit. Rooming-in, where babies stay with mothers, is encouraged in more and more hospitals, since it's an ideal time for parents to get to know their infants and learn the best way of caring for them.

Nurse Yaussy explains, "One of the most exciting moments for me is when I see parents so happy and involved with their child. We call it 'bonding.' Fathers are allowed to carry their baby from the delivery room to the nursery and can give their baby his first bath. It can be a very touching moment and means a lot for the future happiness of the family."

Nurse Yaussy, who works part-time because of family obligations, feels that "it's almost a requirement in obstetrics that the nurse be a mother. Some women have a hard time when they have babies—some don't. When the nurse has been through the experience herself, she can be more understanding and probably has more credibility with her patients."

Nurse Yaussy usually works in postpartum or the nursery, although occasionally she's assigned to labor and delivery. "We practice primary nursing here, and since the census fluctuates so much, I can have as many as ten patients to care for or as few as one. The average is four to five. All deliveries in this hospital are performed by obstetricians— there are no nurse-midwives on staff.

"In the labor room, when a normal delivery is expected, the staff nurse will check the patient every hour. As labor progresses, the checks will come every fifteen minutes, and in some situations, as when special medication is given, the obstetrics nurse does not leave the patient's side. The same nurse who has cared for the mother during labor will also be the one to set up and help with the delivery and will continue to monitor the mother in the recovery room.

"In a normal delivery, mothers and babies usually stay in the hospital for two full days. On the postpartum floor, the nurse is responsible for assisting the mother out of bed for the first time and assessing her condition. Much of the nurse's time on the postpartum unit is spent in teaching the mother about personal care as well as breast feeding, bottle feeding, giving baby a bath, and general parenting skills."

For the nurse assigned to the newborn nursery, there can also be parent teaching. "Recently we had a baby with a cleft palate, and as the nursery nurse, I showed the parents how to feed and care for the child."

As in most nursing care, the usual and routine can quickly become a stressful emergency. Mothers may need caesarean sections (the baby is delivered through an incision in the mother's abdomen and womb). Occasionally, babies are born with birth defects. If the defect is serious and life threatening, the infant is moved to the neonatal intensive care unit. Since most small-sized hospitals, such as the one where Nurse Yaussy works, do not have the day-to-day need for this kind of unit, the seriously ill babies are transferred to a regional center. Most communities follow this practice.

Nurse Yaussy sums up: "To be a good obstetrical nurse requires that you be assertive and not easily flustered. It helps to have some medical and surgical experience beforehand, since some mothers do have other medical problems. And, of course, you must like babies and new mothers. That's usually the easiest part of the job!"

Pediatric Nursing

From infancy until the age of 16, patients receive medical care on a pediatric unit. Margo Cleveland, RN, is a part-time pediatric staff nurse at a sprawling medical center in upstate New York. This is a large unit and is divided into three areas—a pediatric intensive care unit and two medical-surgical pediatric wings. The task-oriented method of nursing is practiced here, and Nurse Cleveland is always responsible for patient care (rather than acting as charge or medication nurse). On the evening shift she cares for between five and ten children, depending on the number of staff members on duty and the census of the unit.

Nurse Cleveland explains her usual duties: "I arrive at three on one of the medical-surgical wings. After reviewing the Kardex and nursing care plans for each of my assigned patients, I listen to report from the day nurse and then immediately go to all my patients, seeing the most ill ones first. I check IVs, dressings, and casts, take vital signs, and assess the general condition of each child. I also check for safety in each room. I make sure the side rails are securely up on all cribs and beds and see that the call lights are within easy reach. There may be treatments before supper, such as diabetic testing. Supper comes early on pediatrics, and the little ones often need help with eating. There's usually a few extra trips to the kitchen for additional food for fussy eaters and hungry teenagers. Food and fluid intake and output is charted hourly for each pediatric patient, and this is done after mealtime.

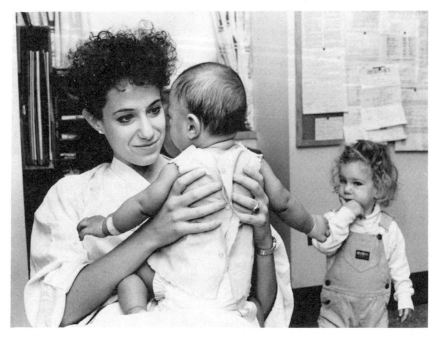

A pediatric nurse holds an infant patient. *(Photo by Irene B. Bayer)*

"Following my supper break, there's usually time to restock patients' rooms with supplies of linen, formula, diapers, sterile dressings, and so on. Then there are dressing changes and bottle feedings. By 7:30, I check and record vital signs on my patients. Snacks are passed out, and the younger children are settled for the night. For youngsters having surgery the next day, there is preop teaching for the child and his parents. The rest of the evening is spent in finishing treatments, straightening up the patients' units, and charting or making notes on each child's progress."

Nurse Cleveland, a diploma graduate, has had wide experience in medical-surgical, emergency room, and operating room nursing as well as pediatrics and school nursing. She feels that an easygoing personality is helpful in pediatrics and that the nurse needs to like children (and their parents) and understand normal growth and development patterns.

Nurse Cleveland admits some frustration in her work: "There's never enough time to rock fussy babies, play with a fun-loving toddler,

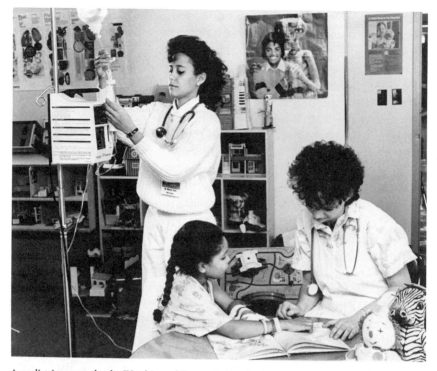

A pediatric nurse checks IV tubing while another pediatric nurse reads a book with a patient. *(Photo by Irene B. Bayer)]*

read a story to a lonesome kid, play a game with a bored preteen or teenager, or have an intelligent conversation with a worried mom or dad. There's hardly enough time to get the simple basics of care done, and I don't like that part of it. It's also upsetting sometimes to work with really sick kids and have to do treatments that are painful. When children are admitted who have been abused by their parents, it can be very sad. You *do* get emotionally involved sometimes.

"The thing that warms my heart, though, is the sight of a smile—no matter how small—on the face of a patient. It doesn't matter if the child is 3 months or 13 years old. That smile makes all my hard work worthwhile."

Other Specialities

Nurses may have specialties within the hospital setting that fall outside the traditional areas described. One example is the nurse who works as a part of an IV team. These nurses circulate through certain areas of the hospital and start all intravenous solutions on patients requiring this type of therapy. In some cases, these nurses may also start blood transfusions.

Moving closer to the administrative department, a nurse may hold a position as ombudsman. It is this person's job to smooth relations between the patient and the hospital. The nurse investigates patient complaints, reports findings, and helps to achieve an equitable agreement between the patient and the hospital.

Finally, a nurse may work as a utilization review coordinator. This nurse is responsible for reviewing the admissions and extended stay of all medicare beneficiaries to determine the medical necessity of such care. The nurse (or nurses) checks patients and their records to gather information for the utilization review committee. It is also this nurse's job to see that the hospital has met its objective of providing high-quality patient care and has efficiently utilized available health facilities and services.

The utilization review nurse spends much of her time reviewing patients' records and talking with doctors. Her position requires that she have considerable knowledge of modern nursing techniques and procedures and knowledge of medical terminology, diagnosis, and methods of treatment. This knowledge is necessary in order to obtain a full understanding of a Medicare patient's need for further hospitalization. This nurse must be able to work and communicate amicably with physicians under what may be stressful situations.

THE NEW SPECIALTIES

Because of increased knowledge and technological advances, health care today is very complex. Hospitals have responded to this complexity by increasing the number of specialized units within their facilities. Units that could only be imagined a generation ago are now standard in most hospitals. Many nurses have carved out exciting careers for themselves in these new fields of specialization.

Critical-Care Nursing

The intensive care unit (ICU) at a 300-bed public hospital in Escondido, California, is an area of the hospital with one of the highest stress levels for patients, families, and health personnel.

This unit is divided into two sections—the first is a six-bed section that's down the hall from an eight-bed ICU that's designed to resemble a fish bowl. The nurses' station is located in the middle, and the patient rooms radiate around this central area. Each room has a wide doorway or a glass panel so that nurses literally do not take their eyes off their patients, even while sitting at the nurses' desk. There is no day or night in this unit and there is no peace for either patients or nurses here.

Paula White has been a nurse in the unit for eight and a half years and is now an assistant nurse manager. Before that, she worked for one year in an intensive care unit in a small community hospital and for one year in an ICU in a large, highly specialized hospital. In her present position, White works four ten-hour day shifts per week (5:30 a.m. to 4:00 p.m.) and admittedly enjoys the stress and challenge of working in this specialty. She explains the type of patient that is cared for in the unit: "If a patient needs a ventilator to help him breathe, regardless of his diagnosis, he is transferred to intensive care. Some other patients we care for are serious postoperative cases (including patients with open heart surgery), plus patients suffering from drug overdose, serious internal bleeding, and trauma (some large hospitals have separate trauma units or separate neurological or pulmonary units). Patients usually stay in our ICU for three days, although neurological patients may stay for up to two weeks.

"There are normally five RNs and a ward clerk assigned to the day shift and four on the night shift. That usually works out to two patients for every nurse, although nurses frequently have to work one-on-one with a patient because of the complex equipment and close monitoring that is required.

"In the ICU there's a lot of equipment crammed into a small space and there's always a cluttered look about the place. There are monitors at each bedside and a main monitor at the nurse's station. There's a lot of bells and buzzers and bleeping alarms that add to the busyness and tension of the unit.

"In this hospital we see a lot of patients with trauma injuries. A young person, for example, may be thrown from a car and he's brought to the emergency room with a fracture of the pelvis and femur. This is not the patient's most serious problem, though. What happens is that, because of a head injury, the brain swells and there's increased intracranial pressure. This becomes a medical emergency and the neurosurgeon will do whatever is necessary to try to prevent permanent brain damage. He may drain cerebrospinal fluid by putting in a line or he may have to perform surgery to relieve the pressure.

"The patient who is suffering from a head trauma is always brought to our unit. Because there are usually breathing difficulties, a tube is passed through his nose, mouth, or through an incision in the neck [called a tracheostomy] and the patient is hooked up to the ventilator, which will mechanically breathe for him. There is usually a problem with temperature control so the patient may have to be warmed up or cooled down. Generally, the temperature is kept low so that oxygen demand is less. We usually start two or three IV lines. Medications are given intravenously, and since some medicines are not compatible with others, there has to be more than one line.

"An arterial line is usually put in place so that we can get immediate blood pressure readings and readily take arterial blood samples. A nasogastric tube is passed through the nose and into the stomach. This keeps the stomach empty, prevents vomiting and aspiration of stomach contents, and keeps a check on bleeding in that area. There may be a pressure line in the head, EKG lines are always hooked up to measure cardiac rhythms, and there is undoubtedly a Foley catheter in place since the patient has no bladder control."

"The patient can hardly be seen for all the spaghettilike lines that are coming from his body and going to the various machines that keep him alive or monitor his condition. These monitors go off if there's a malfunction or even if the patient makes a wrong move in bed."

"For a patient such as this, the intensive care nurse would be checking the patient's blood pressure and neurological status every fifteen minutes until they were stable. In order for the ventilator to work properly, she may have to suction lung secretions every twenty minutes. There would be round-the-clock medications, and the nurse must know the action of these so well that she can pick up any untoward effects immediately. In a neurological patient, the temperature must be taken at least every hour and the nurse may need to bathe the patient, give mouth care, and change the bed linens frequently. Every two hours, sometimes every hour, the patient is turned and positioned with pillows. This is done to prevent complications and goes on day and night.

"All the work that the nurse does for the patient must be documented in the chart. As the neuro patient stabilizes, we may do range-of-motion exercises, take measures to prevent foot drop, and we may begin tube feedings through the nasogastric tube.

"If all this sounds physically exhausting, it usually is. Sometimes I don't sit down all night. But usually the greater exhaustion comes from the emotional involvement. I may care for a child who's been in an automobile accident and is the same age as one of my children. Or I may have to explain and give comfort to family members. And nurses are often the ones who have to sort out conflicting orders or pin down doctors to find out their plans for the patient."

Nurse White continues: "It's estimated that the average ICU patient has fifty people passing through his room every day. He may have four or five physicians caring for him. There is little control over the environment and things can get very hectic. An X-ray machine may be wheeled into the small unit or in case of a 'code' [a patient has stopped breathing or lost a palpable pulse] there may be as many as ten people around the bedside trying to resuscitate the patient.

"One of the biggest pressures for me is staffing. There is only so much that one nurse can do. I don't know of any ICU nurse who can laugh off or ignore poor care. Most of us try to treat patients as we would like to be treated. You're always saying, 'I have to do this ... and this ... and this.' I know that if the patient doesn't do well because I've messed up, I'll have to deal with it. So that pressure is always there. I remember one of the nurses broke down and cried because there was no one to help her turn a patient. Of course it seems silly to cry about that. But it shows the kind of tension we work under.

"You have to set priorities in this specialty and have to have high personal standards and stick with them. You have to be a fast thinker but also flexible. Because of the physical demands, mostly young nurses work in ICU. Most are fairly aggressive and will fight for proper patient care.

"For a student interested in this specialty, I would suggest a strong background in anatomy and physiology with the understanding that learning must never stop and must be the nurse's responsibility."

White, who is a graduate of an AD program, feels that learning the scientific principles while in school is very important. "The skills will come later—on the job—but the background has to be there first.

"Critical care nursing is usually very satisfying work. The nurse intervenes in a crisis situation and the patient is often saved—and may even return to a normal life—because of your efforts. I like what I'm doing and wouldn't want to work anyplace else."

Other areas where critical-care nursing is practiced are the neonatal (newborn infants) unit, pediatric intensive care unit, and the coronary care unit. These units are all similar to the ICU just described in that the pace is fast, a crisis is always just minutes away, and the patient receives the absolute best care that medicine and nursing can offer.

A coronary care unit is designed to provide care for those who have

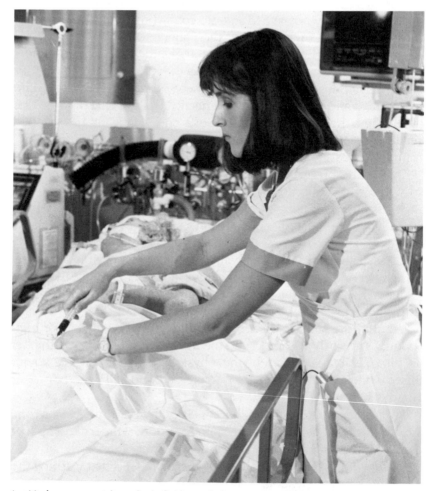

A critical care nurse takes a body fluid sample from a patient. *(Photo by Harriet Gans)*

had or are suspected of having had recent heart attacks. There's generally less equipment in this unit. Patients may receive intravenous and oxygen therapy and are hooked up to heart monitoring machines, but in coronary care the emphasis is on rest for the patient, so things are kept as quiet as possible. Rooms are more likely to be partitioned off and privacy is allowed. There is differentiation between day and night, and meals are served. As one critical-care nurse said, "In coronary care, there may be more sitting for the nurse but it's like sitting on a time bomb. Cardiac rhythms have to be watched and things can change, at a moment's notice, from peace and quiet to high tension."

Burn Center

An 8-year-old tow-headed boy scoots around the hospital corridor, weaving back and forth among the doctors, nurses, and patients and giving a friendly "Hiya" to all he meets. He holds a disposable syringe—minus the needle—in one hand. The syringe is filled with water, and every now and again he squirts some of the liquid into his mouth. It's a hospital version of a squirt gun and gives respite on a hot summer day.

In spite of the normality of his play, though, it's obvious there's something unusual about this child. Instead of a shirt, he wears a white netting vest, and gauze strips show underneath the net. And the way the boy moves his legs is something between a hobble and a limp. Just below his cutoff pants, you can see that the spindly legs are scarred from burns.

This 8-year-old boy has been a patient in the burn unit at the University of California at San Diego Medical Center for several months. He's one of ten burn victims who range in age from 1 year to over 60. The unit can accommodate up to fourteen patients and serves the areas of San Diego and Imperial counties. As much as these patients are the same, they are all different, too. And the burn unit itself is a very different place to work.

Alice Kayuha, RN, has worked on the unit for seven years and has been director for one year. She explains the relatively new concept of burn treatment: "During World War II, burn victims were treated as surgical patients, and many were taken to Brooks Institute at Fort Sam Houston in Texas. Primary research was done there, and it was discovered that the burn victim was a very special patient. A burn is a total body injury—it involves physical considerations (shock, fluid replacement, infection, reconstruction) and psychological needs (adjustment to disfigurement). Because burns were seen as more than a surgical problem, a team concept evolved as a more efficient approach to treatment of burn patients.

"In this unit, for example, our team consists of two attending surgeons, members of the house staff (interns and residents), a physician assistant, the patient care coordinator or clinical nurse specialist, physical and occupational therapists, a dietician, a pharmacist, the director of the skin bank, and the mental health team. The mental health team is made up of a psychiatrist, psychologist, and psychiatric social worker. They work with patients, family, and staff. Once a week, there's a meeting of this whole group. And because we're a university hospital, there are teaching rounds with the patients three times a week. As we need them, we call in specialists from other areas of the hospital—all the reconstruction work, for example, is done by a plastic surgeon."

The Medical Center burn unit is a regional center and is self-contained. Another approach to treatment of burn victims is a smaller hospital burn unit that serves only the hospital district. Some hospitals have "burn beds" that are used as the need arises, and in one Florida hospital burn patients are housed throughout the hospital and are treated by a burn team that moves through different hospital areas to care for each burn victim.

The typical burn patient at the Medical Center has burns covering 30 to 40 percent of the body. The usual stay is measured in months rather than weeks. Nurses on this unit are able to develop long-term relationships with their patients.

According to Director Kayuha, "the body surface that's burned doesn't always predict the rate of recovery. Many times elderly patients have only a 20 percent burn, but the shock to the body sends them into congestive heart failure or renal failure. In other words, a burn is a total body injury and can affect all organs."

The San Diego area burn victim is admitted directly to the Medical Center unit and is placed in the burn intensive care unit. As in other ICUs, there is much sophisticated equipment—respirators, IVs, tubes and lines of all sorts. "We're concerned with septic shock, prevention of infection, fluid replacement. The patient is very seriously ill and the nurse working in this unit is under considerable stress as she performs life-saving tasks. Once the patient is stabilized and no longer requires constant care, he is transferred to the special care area and the philosophy of his treatment completely changes. Where before the patient's role was a passive one, the nurse now insists on independence as the long road to recovery begins. Even though the patient may not have skin on his legs, we insist he must walk. And even though it's painful to do so, we insist he feed himself.

"Then there's the daily bath. This is done in the treatment area, and a group of nurses is also assigned there. The patient is lifted by a hammocklike hydraulic device into a large vat of warm solution. Special abrasive material is used by nurses to scrub dead material from the skin.

"The bath and dressing changes are painful to the patient and never a pleasure. He may scream out in pain, and this is a difficult time for the nurse too."

Nurse Kayuha continues: "We had two young boys here one time and they were playing 'doctor.' The nurse was the patient and was put to bed. The role play was very interesting. They got the biggest syringe they could find to give their 'patient' a 'shot,' and when it came time for the bath treatment, the boys told their nurse patient, 'Now, we're going to give you some medicine so this won't hurt. But of course it does hurt—it always hurts—they're just kidding when they say it doesn't.'"

Twenty-six full-time RNs work around the clock on the burn unit. There are graduates of AD, diploma, and baccalaureate programs. There are a few LPNs, but they are being phased out. The RNs rotate between intensive care, special care, and treatment. They're also responsible for working in the out-patient burn clinics two days a week.

"If a nurse can stay here for six months, she usually will last at least two years. We have quite a number of nurses who have worked here for four to five years, but the work is physically and emotionally hard. A burn unit nurse has to be flexible enough to shift gears in a matter of minutes. She can be sitting around waiting for something to happen and within minutes be at full work force. We rotate our nurses through the three areas to change the pace and eliminate some of the stressors. In the ICU burn area, there are many complicated tasks to perform— that's similar to other ICUs. But in our ICU the turnover is not as fast and so the pace is not as frantic. In the special care area, the emphasis is on rehabilitation. That requires patience and understanding. The sort of nurse who usually does well here is the kind who likes medicine over surgery and has had some medical experience. She should be interested in burn patients rather than in just a nursing 'job.' And she should like a lot of patient contact and long-term care.

"There are certain problems that nurses encounter here that are peculiar to the unit. A nurse does very little for her patient that doesn't involve pain. A nurse's instinct is to relieve pain—not make it worse. But if the patient isn't turned every two hours, he'll get pneumonia. And there are the baths and the walking—it's all painful.

"Burns cause disfigurement of the body. A nurse can't help but think with a child, 'What will it be like for him when he's 16 and trying to make friends? How will he cope?' We had one man in here who had severe facial burns—those are the worst. At first we thought he wouldn't live, but he did survive and we got to know him very well. It was almost as though someone had pulled a nylon stocking over his face—all his features were pulled out of shape and distorted. His nose was gone and there were only two holes left. There were only patches of hair on his head. He was very strong and was here for a long time. After a time, we nurses didn't notice the disfigurement. It's like there are two people—the inside person and the outside person. The inside person was the one we got to know. But other people—strangers mostly—would stare and point. And the nurses resented that. We became very protective—probably too much so. This is one of the issues that must be dealt with. Many people working on this unit learn to have different views on appearance after working here. They don't see it as being that important, even though society says it is.

"The worst time for a nurse is when a patient dies. That may come after the patient has been on the unit for three months and the nurse knows that in all that time she never gave that patient a moment of peace.

"But there are good parts to the job—probably the best is the long-term relationships you have with patients. They stay on the unit for an extended time and then they're followed at the out-patient clinic. And the staff on a burn unit are very special people. They work well together. Usually they have a good sense of humor—I suppose that's part of the coping mechanism—and they're very supportive of one another. We're a good solid bunch—very interested in our patients and each other."

Dialysis Nurse

John Stephens sits in a recliner chair reading his newspaper. He appears quite relaxed and jokes with the dialysis nurse as she adjusts the tubes that connect the shunt on Stephen's left forearm to the machine that keeps him alive. Three times a week, for the rest of his life, John Stephens will be attached to this life-support machine. He is one of 90,886 people in the United States who rely on kidney dialysis to regulate chemical levels in their blood.

When a patient's kidneys fail, he or she is no longer able to separate and remove the waste products and excess fluid from the bloodstream. Medical science can provide two life-saving solutions—one is kidney transplantation and the other is dialysis. Patients who receive dialysis suffer from either acute renal failure or chronic end-stage renal disease.

There are several methods of dialysis, the oldest being *hemodialysis*, which is a process whereby blood is circulated through a machine and "washed" clean of fluid wastes. Hemodialysis can be carried out in a hospital-type setting or in a patient's home. In *continuous ambulatory peritoneal dialysis* (CAPD), fluid flows into the patient's abdomen and drains out (at the same time pulling off toxins). The patient does the CAPD himself and is free to walk about and pursue other activities while being dialyzed.

Nurses who care for the growing number of dialysis patients are called dialysis nurses. Pamela Thompson, RN, of Miami, Florida, has been a dialysis nurse since 1968, when she worked in one of the twelve original units funded by a U.S. Public Health Service grant. These first dialysis facilities were home-training units that taught the patient and his or her spouse or partner how to perform hemodialysis at home. Afterwards, Thompson established a home-training unit in a local hospital that taught patients from out of state as well as patients from Central and South America and the Caribbean. This unit progressed to a ten-station acute/chronic dialysis facility treating the sickest chronic patients in the community as well as acutely ill patients with renal failure. Thompson has also been administrator of a thirteen-station proprietary out-patient dialysis center. In this post, she was responsible for the total business and clinical operation of the unit. At the present time, Nurse Thompson is director of nursing at the twenty-eight station out-patient Dade Dialysis Center, which is part of Florida's end-stage renal disease network (there are thirty-two such networks in the country).

In her present job, Thompson is responsible for directing and evaluating patient care policies, maintaining quality care, and sharing the fiscal responsibility with other administrators to make the unit cost effective.

Thompson's career has paralleled the history of dialysis nursing, and she is quick to point out the many fields that are now open for nurses within this specialty: "There is career development for all aspects of nursing: clinical, education, and administrative. The dialysis nurse can work in a chronic unit or an acute unit, she can direct a training program for new staff, or she can train patients for home dialysis. In addition, the nurse can perform hemodialysis or supervise continuous ambulatory peritoneal dialysis. The nurse can also work in a hospital that performs transplant operations or can work for an industry that manufactures dialysis supplies and equipment. In this role, nursing duties involve providing in-service education to staff nurses who use the equipment. Dialysis nursing is a rapidly growing specialty with every-changing improved techniques and treatment programs."

As with most nursing fields, the beginning position for a dialysis nurse is on the staff level. Where does a staff dialysis nurse work and what does she do?

The treatment area that accommodates one patient is called a station—the number of stations determines the size of the dialysis unit. Stations are generally small and cramped. In an area of slightly over

100 square feet, there is a large recliner chair for the patient, the hemodialysis machine, and other necessary equipment. Patients are usually treated three times per week; each treatment lasts for four hours. In most units, families are discouraged from staying with the patient during dialysis to prevent crowding and to provide privacy for other patients.

One nurse described the dialysis unit as a "factorylike ICU." Two patient shifts are usually dialyzed in a day. The same faces, the same routine—this is the "factory" part. Dialyzing a patient, however, requires such critical-care skills as detection of heart arrhythmias, emergency treatment of low blood pressure, and administration of CPR. In Nurse Thompson's words, "working in a dialysis unit may be described as hours and hours of routine interspersed with moments of sheer panic."

Equipment breakdown must be recognized and corrected by the nurse. Many units employ technicians to maintain and repair equipment, but the nurse must also be familiar with the mechanical functions of the machines.

In a chronic dialysis unit, one staff RN is usually responsible for the care of three patients. In an acute unit, the patient-nurse ratio is normally one to one. In both areas, the nurse is responsible for evaluating the patient's status before, during, and after dialysis and planning the treatment to meet the patient's goals for the day. The staff RN evaluates fluid and electrolyte balance, signs and symptoms of complications of end-stage renal disease, signs and symptoms of dialysis-related complications, laboratory status, and response to the prescribed medication.

The nurse has a primary role in both the short-term and long-term treatment plan. Most dialysis patients are seen by a physician one to three times a week. Physicians, however, are not continually present in the dialysis unit. Therefore, the nurse functions independently with appropriate physician consultation by telephone. The dialysis nurse also works closely with other members of the health team, including the social worker, dietician, home health nurse, and occupational therapist.

The nurse instructs the patient and the family in such areas as hygiene and care of the access site. In hemodialysis, the surgeon makes an opening into the patient's vein and an artery and connects the two openings with plastic tubing. This method produces a *shunt* and is usually done on the forearm. The tubing lies outside the arm and is kept in place with a bandage. Another method is to connect an artery and vein under the skin. This is called a *fistula*. Blood travels to the kidney machine and returns by means of needles inserted in the fistula.

In CAPD, the lining of the abdomen (or peritoneum) is used to separate waste products. In this type of dialysis, a plastic tube is inserted through the abdominal wall just below the navel and fixed in place. A plastic bag, filled with a solution similar to that used in the kidney machine, is connected to the tube. The solution then flows from the bag into the abdominal cavity. The empty bag is folded up and placed beneath the patient's clothing. After four to six hours, the empty bag is reconnected to the plastic tube. The solution, now containing the waste products separated by the peritoneum, flows back into the bag, and a new bag is attached. This process is repeated every day. There are many advantages to CAPD, but the most serious disadvantage is the risk of infecting the peritoneum. For this reason, patient hygiene is very important.

The nurse also instructs the patient and the family on proper nutrition, on action, dose, and side effects of medications, and on other areas of health management. The nurse is a listener who is often in a therapeutic friendship role with the patient. Often patients tell their most intimate problems to the nursing staff before confiding in the physician. It is the nurse's responsibility to aid the patient in getting the assistance or information required.

In a unit that trains patients and their spouses or partners to perform dialysis in the home, the training nurse is the primary nurse to interact with the patient. The nurse must teach the patient to perform a dialysis independently, troubleshoot medical and equipment problems, and understand and adhere to the prescribed medical, dietary, and social regimens. The patient and partner must know as much about dialysis as a patient care technician. After the patient dialyzes in the home, the nurse visits to ensure quality of care and evaluate the patient's overall status.

According to Nurse Thompson, "the best part of the job is the close interpersonal relationships established with the patient and family. It's also satisfying to serve as an important functioning member of the health care team and have the opportunity to learn in a rapidly growing and innovative field.

"The most difficult aspect of the job also involves the close relationships established with a patient and the difficult task of watching that patient suffer with complications or fail and die. It is like having a friend die and everyone in the unit may go through a grieving process. Often group sessions allow the staff to vent their frustrations and grief.

"The job is generally more taxing emotionally than physically, although the nurse tends to spend most of the shift on her feet with little time to actually sit and work.

"The pressures of the job, other than patient relationships and occasional complications, are usually the result of attempts to follow a time schedule and get all patients on and off the machine on time. Patients are extremely anxious to get on the machine and become very upset when delayed in any manner. Time factors are important in the management of the unit, as several shifts of patients are usually dialyzed during one staff shift, and in order to treat all patients without the use of staff overtime, schedules must be adhered to closely. Other pressures are created by a staff group that works in a confined area. Harmony must be created by a sincere effort to get along with others, much like the situation in an ICU or operating room.

"It is impossible for an RN to work effectively in a dialysis unit without additional formal training because of the specialized nature of the job. My background is BSN with six months of coronary care experience. Most dialysis nurses don't have a baccalaureate degree, and it's not a requirement to do a good job. With the increasing demand for nurses in the Miami area and the shortage of nurses, we have relaxed our previous desire for a nurse with critical care experience to one with medical-surgical background. Nurses are taught dialysis in a one-to-three-month course consisting of on-the-job training supplemented with classroom teaching.

"Prospective dialysis nurses can work in a facility as a technician during school breaks or after school to learn the skills involved in giving a treatment. They can also learn first-hand how a dialysis unit operates and be a valuable trained employee when hired as an RN."

Oncology Nursing

Pam Crone is a registered nurse in an 18-bed oncology (cancer) unit in an average-sized general hospital in the area of Seattle, Washington. She's worked in the unit for eight years and frankly admits that "as a student, I never dreamed I would work with cancer patients—I always wanted to care for the babies in the nursery. But that can get boring. Working with cancer patients puts your own life in a different perspective. The rewards can be very meaningful but it takes a certain level of maturity. An oncology nurse has to feel comfortable about people dying and has to be in touch with her own feelings."

In the unit where Nurse Crone works, there is an all-RN staff and primary nursing is practiced. On her unit, each nurse is responsible for the care of four patients. Because of this, she gets to know her patients and their families very well. Patients may stay on the unit for several days to several months. They may be discharged and then readmitted, but the same nurse follows them all the way through their hospitalization.

"We only work with four physicians and we get to know them well, too. We're a close group and members of the team get a lot of support from one another. Once a week, we have a group meeting with the psychiatrist to deal with our work-related problems. To be an oncology nurse means constantly going through the grief process. We nurses don't just lose one person when a patient dies. We work closely with families and become their friends. We lose that relationship too when the patient dies.

"Working with cancer patients involves much more than relieving physical pain and suffering. It's fairly easy to control that. And in carrying out a program of chemotherapy, it's not hard to read directions for administering drugs and to watch for adverse reactions and signs of sepsis [infection]. In oncology nursing, it's the emotional side of patient care that's the most challenging. You work with patients and families to help them accept the diagnosis and help them plan for the days ahead. It's that terrible fear of the unknown and working through the grieving process.

"The important skills for an oncology nurse lie in effective communication and being a patient advocate. A doctor may visit his patient, for example, and in the course of conversation the patient may say, 'What did my gallbladder exam show?' The doctor will answer, 'Don't worry about that—we'll take care of it.' For one reason or another, the patient does not pursue the point with the doctor but will say to his nurse, 'Dr. Hill never answers my questions fully. He says not to worry about it, but I do worry.' So the next time Dr. Hill visits his patient, the nurse is also there and she explains to the doctor, 'Mr. Jones would like more specific details about the gallbladder exam.' The nurse will listen to Dr. Hill's explanation and observe Mr. Jones. If she doesn't feel that her patient is satisfied, she'll try to help clarify the point.

"Still another time, a patient might have completed three or four different therapies and there's still no remission. The patient is exhausted and ready to be done with it. But the doctor might not want to give up and might want to continue with another therapy. The nurse's role is to talk with the doctor and find out what's going on with him emotionally—to find out why he can't change the focus of his treatment plan."

Nurse Crone explains that there is a wide variation in oncology nursing. "On our unit, for example, we have much leeway in ordering certain drugs and participating in the patient's treatment program. In other units, this is not true. We have low staff turnover here and few people leave because of burnout. In one eastern hospital, they improved job satisfaction by rotating nurses between the three areas of out-patient clinic, hospital and data collection. The nurses spend six weeks on each of these units."

Although Nurse Crone works in a special unit within a general hospital, some oncology nurses work in large cancer centers where bone marrow transplants are done and experimental treatments are performed. Some hospitals care exclusively for children who have cancer.

These centers are important for the advancement of research and for patient treatment when more sophisticated equipment is needed. But day-to-day care usually takes place in a hospital near the patient's home. For this reason, many hospitals are making special provisions for cancer patients. Part of this includes the use of nurses who specialize in oncology nursing.

Enterostomal Therapy

There are approximately 2,000 registered nurses who specialize exclusively in enterostomal therapy, and in terms of numbers, that may not seem very large. But in terms of job satisfaction and benefits to the health care team, enterostomal therapists (ETs) are an impressive group.

As Kay Ascani, RN, ET, of Washington, D.C., explains, "I often hear from the health care givers that I work with, 'ETs have *got* to be a special kind of people.' Then, too, in my orientation classes, someone always asks me about schools for enterostomal therapy training. They say, 'I think I'd like that type of nursing specialty. What are the requirements?'"

An enterostomal therapist is a registered nurse with a baccalaureate degree who has completed a six-to-eight-week intensive postgraduate clinical course and is then certified to care for the specialized needs of patients with ostomy-type surgery. In these operations, which have increased appreciably in number over the past twenty years, portions of the patient's intestinal or urinary tract are removed or diverted and an artificial opening, or *stoma*, is constructed through the abdominal wall to allow for passage of urine or feces. The waste products drain into a special pouch that fits over the artificial opening (except for the continent ileostomy patient, in which case the pouch is internal). In addition to helping patients who have had ostomy surgery, ETs also manage difficult wounds in those areas requiring containment of excretion. Some are involved with the prevention and treatment of skin ulcers (including diabetic ulcers and bedsores) as well as tissue trauma management and incontinence (bowel and bladder training).

This may not sound like glamorous work, but the services that ETs perform are absolutely essential and most rewarding. They enjoy considerable authority and respect among members of the health care team.

Daily schedules must be flexible in order to accommodate the unexpected and various daily requests. Kay Ascani, a full-time enterostomal therapist at Washington's Greater Southeast Community Hospital, described a day in her life as an ET: "I arrive at the office at 8:00 a.m. and usually spend the first hour or so preparing schedules for continuing nursing education, writing care plans, requisitioning supplies, and answering telephone calls from patients with problems. I check on those who have been discharged and answer letters and calls from community health nurses, physicians, or other hospital personnel.

"At 9:30, I start daily rounds, visiting all ostomy patients and checking decubital ulcers, wound problems, and following up on physician-requested consultations. I may, in conjunction with the dietary department, discuss nutritional concerns for malnourished patients and those patients scheduled for or receiving chemotherapy or radiation.

"If my patients are approaching discharge, I may meet with families for teaching purposes or may meet with the continuing care coordinator for hospital follow-up. Some days I work with patients who have already been discharged but are having ostomy problems. A good part of my time is spent teaching the staff nurse as well as the patient at the bedside.

"My responsibilities are indefinable at times, but a holistic approach to the patient is the key to success, and I do what needs to be done to provide the patient with quality care. Late in the afternoon I prepare my schedule for the following day, after attending to those patient problems that surfaced on rounds."

Kay Ascani has considerable flexibility in her work. She has opportunities to pursue research (with supervisory support) and to attend seminars and conferences. One important example of the autonomy that ETs enjoy is their opportunity (as well as responsibility) to mark the site where the stoma will be located after the patient's surgery. When patients are admitted with ulcers, she assesses, plans, and implements a care plan after obtaining a physician's order. She may also photograph the area in order to record the patient's progress.

Ascani is a member of the hospital geriatric team and provides the nursing assessment as it applies to her expertise. She also teaches a six-week ostomy and ward management course that involves classroom instruction, rounds, and preparation of care plans. This provides a resource nurse on each unit of the hospital.

As for the demands of the job, Ascani feels it is most challenging mentally and emotionally, although considerable physical energy is expended on daily rounds when working with patients. For Ascani, some of the difficulties of the job involve losing patients, to whom she has become very attached, to terminal illness and working with those who are unable to accept their change in body image.

"A good enterostomal nurse should be patient oriented and capable of functioning well with a holistic approach to health care," says Nurse Ascani. "The nurse should be responsible and conscientious and a self-starter (that is, not need supervision). She must be emotionally stable and comfortable with the patient and his family. An ET provides support and security while maintaining and encouraging the patient's sense of humor. To sum up, the nurse who does well in this specialty is generally extroverted and has a deep sense of commitment and concern for others."

There are twelve approved courses in the United States that graduate about 400 enterostomal therapists per year. The schools have long waiting lists. Applicants must be baccalaureate RNs with two years of clinical experience, must have at least two endorsements from physicians attesting to their eligibility, and must ideally be sponsored by a hospital with an ET position available (the last, however, is not mandatory).

Although the basic responsibilities of all ETs are similar, some also work in treatment rooms or assist with colonoscopys (examination of the colon) in addition to their ET duties. Some nurses service more than one hospital.

Kay Ascani is a 1940 graduate of the Lenox Hill Hospital Nursing School in New York City. For twenty-six years, she spent time raising a family of eight children and occasionally worked as a volunteer in military hospitals. In 1966, Nurse Ascani took a refresher course and worked for three years as a medical-surgical staff nurse at the Veterans Administration Center in Dayton, Ohio. Moving to the Washington, D.C. area in 1969, she took a position as staff nurse on an 80-bed medical-surgical unit. After several years she was promoted to assistant head nurse, and then in 1973 she became head nurse of this unit. In

1975, she took the enterostomal therapy course and since then has been the enterostomal therapist at the Community Hospital. Ascani has written many articles for the ostomy newsletter and makes presentations at educational workshops.

Her advice for someone interested in a career as an ET? "Spend time with an enterostomal therapist in a hospital setting and find out if you would enjoy this type of nursing. Write to ET schools and select one with good training. Get on their waiting list. Finally, approach the nursing service in the hospital where you work and see if there would be a position available after you finish school. If this isn't successful, then investigate other areas—such as the Veterans Administration or community health agencies—and see if they are seeking enterostomal therapists."

The Journal of Enterostomal Therapy frequently advertises job opportunities for enterostomal therapists. It's a new nursing specialty and the future will be exciting as the specialty continues to grow and expand into many areas of research and development.

THE TREND TO SHORTER HOSPITAL STAYS

Hospitalization is the most costly way to provide health care. This is an alarming fact for consumers, insurance companies, and the federal government.

In an effort to hold down costs, in 1983 the federal government instituted a new plan to reduce hospital stays for Medicare patients (Medicare is a federal insurance program for the elderly and disabled). The plan is called the diagnostic related groups (DRG) system. Under this plan, Medicare categorizes patients' conditions into disease groups and will pay only a certain amount for each hospital admission. What this means for most Medicare patients (who comprise 40 percent of all hospital patients) is that their hospital stays are shorter and they leave the hospital not fully recuperated. For those patients who need simple surgical procedures (such as cataract surgery), the surgery may not be done in a hospital at all but on an outpatient basis.

The effect of DRGs on most hospitals is that fewer patients are admitted and those who do occupy beds are sicker and require more complex nursing care. Hospitals have found themselves in the position of having to lower costs and, at the same time, provide more intensive care for sicker patients. It's been a challenge.

Because of DRGs, many hospitals have had to cut budgets and, in some cases, freeze wages and lay off personnel. On the positive side,

DRGs have provided nurses with an opportunity to have a greater impact on delivery of nursing care in and out of the hospital. Nursing care, and the cost of this care, has been under increased scrutiny. The value and importance of such care has clearly been documented.

Another change that has affected hospital stays is the growing popularity of HMOs (health maintenance organizations), PPOs (preferred provider organizations) and IPAs (independent practice associations).

HMOs provide full health services to members for a fixed, prepaid fee. All necessary care is provided without additional cost to the member. Since there is an incentive to keep costs down, HMOs emphasize prevention of illness and early treatment before costly hospitalization is required. Most HMOs own their own hospitals, but some contract for inpatient care with other institutions in the community.

There are certain characteristics that are typical of HMOs and they affect how health care is provided. Kaiser, the largest HMO in the country, attains its greatest savings by keeping patients out of the hospital. This doesn't mean that Kaiser patients are healthier or receive less care than patients in traditional health plans. What it does mean is that hospitalization is avoided by performing many surgical procedures and almost all tests on an outpatient basis.

In addition, there's no economic incentive for Kaiser physicians to do unnecessary surgery because they receive the same salary no matter how many times they operate.

Other ways that Kaiser reduces costs is by using nurse practitioners (and physicians' assistants) as primary health care providers and utilizing nurse anesthetists (with supervision by MD anesthesiologists) in surgery.

Finally, health education has proven to be an effective way to reduce illness and treat chronic illness at Kaiser. Programs ranging from stress reduction to dieting, from stopping smoking to management of high blood pressure are often managed by nurses and have proven to be effective.

As recently as ten years ago, there was considerable resistance to the concept of HMOs (particularly by the medical community). Today, however, because of financial restraints in all health care institutions, much of the HMO philosophy is being accepted as a necessary change.

In addition to HMOs, there are other health care choices that are now available to the consumer which also reduce hospital stays. In independent practice associations, or IPAs, physicians band together and contract with hospitals to provide medical service at a fixed rate, then offer a prepaid group plan to employee groups. Unlike HMOs, however, doctors belonging to IPAs usually treat both fee-for-service patients and prepaid group patients.

Still another alternative is the PPO (preferred provider organization), in which medical costs are held down by charging less, using only certain facilities, and relying less on costly treatments such as surgery.

Because of all of these cost-containing measures, patients now go to the hospital less often and stay for a shorter time.

CHAPTER 7

Nonhospital Careers

Many general hospitals provide limited, short-term care for the patient requiring psychiatric or rehabilitative management. But for many patients, such therapy occurs in a separate psychiatric or rehabilitation center. For this reason, these specialties, as well as geriatric nursing, will be examined in this chapter.

PSYCHIATRIC NURSING

Before becoming a head nurse, Cathy Anastas Mitchell, RN, worked as a staff nurse in a large (1,000-bed) private psychiatric hospital in the suburbs of Boston. In this position she worked a rotating schedule of days and evenings and was usually assigned to the 12-to-15-year-old children's unit (this is one of four units in the children's center). There were usually fifteen patients on the unit.

Most of the young people on this unit are not physically ill. Unlike treatment for patients who have a specific physical ailment, the psychiatric course of therapy is not as fixed. Treatment consists of learning new insights about one's self and one's relationships. The psychiatrist works on an individual basis and in group therapy with the patients. The psychiatric social worker works with the patient's family and community agencies. The nurse on the unit works with patients on a day-to-day basis as they move through their activities. She monitors and observes the patient's behavior, writes care plans, dispenses medications, and participates in treatment programs. As a supervisor to the aides or counselors on the unit, she teaches basic theories, approaches, and communication skills.

"In psychiatry, more than any other health field, the roles of social worker, psychiatrist, psychologist and nurse often overlap," says Anastas Mitchell. "An experienced psychiatric nurse often has more responsibility and autonomy than other hospital staff nurses. There's also a more open exchange between nurses and doctors."

Anastas Mitchell describes a "typical day": "For the day shift, we arrive at seven. We wear street clothes and that's true of most of the personnel. Usually there's another RN and four to five counselors (aides) on staff. We get report from the night nurse on what has happened in the previous sixteen hours. We find who needs priority attention—for example, who's in seclusion or who was violent. Next, I visit each room and talk to the patients to get a sense of what the day will be like. After the patients have had breakfast—either in the cafeteria or on the unit—we have an 8:30 community meeting in the day room. All personnel—psychiatrists, social workers, and nursing

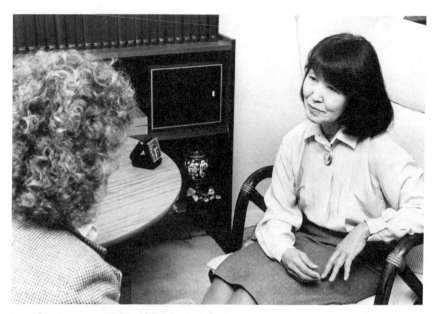

A psychiatric nurse counsels a patient. *(Photo by Irene B. Bayer)*

staff—and patients attend this half-hour meeting. Then the young people go to school at a building adjacent to the hospital. They're in class from 9:00 to 12:00 and from 12:30 to 2:00 although there's often a crisis at the school that the nurse must resolve—and not every child goes to school. From 9:00 to 11:00, there is a team meeting where each patient is discussed. As an out-growth of this, care plans are continually changed, and this is the nurse's responsibility."

Anastas Mitchell described one typical incident with a 14-year-old male patient. "Tom was in the hospital because of family problems and depression, but he usually was a relaxed and talkative boy who responded well to the nurses. One day, I noticed him pacing in the hall. He looked nervous and seemed cautious. I asked him if something was bothering him and he wouldn't answer. So I said, 'Well, if you do decide you want to talk about it, I'm here to listen. I'm available.' Tom went to his room but five minutes later he was back and said, 'Listen, Cath, I have to talk to you. I did something I don't usually do and I don't feel good about it.'

"'What happened?'

"'I ripped off somebody and I feel bad but I don't want to give it back.'

"'What is it that you took, Tom?'

"'A toy soldier.'

"'Can I see it? It must be pretty neat.'"

Tom showed Cathy the toy.

"That's a neat soldier all right. Whose is it?"

"I got it at school—it belongs to the teacher. I want to keep it but I don't know. I feel bad about this."

"How do you think you could make it right?"

"Maybe I could talk to the teacher. You know? Maybe you could come with me?"

Cathy and Tom went to the school and explained the situation to the teacher. After much discussion, she let Tom keep the soldier. By bringing the situation out in the open, Tom was able to resolve his problem and feel good about himself.

"As you can see, there's nothing terribly unusual about this episode. It could happen with any 'normal' teen-ager. The difference is that Tom does have trouble coping or he wouldn't be a patient here. Also, my response to him was consistent with his treatment plan.

"The best part about working here is seeing the growth and progress with these young people and their families. It's very gratifying when the kids get better and are able to return home. The bad part is that, because of staffing cut-backs, the demands on the nurses are greater than they've ever been. This can create problems in supervising the patients. One young man choked me and it took four men to subdue him. Eventually he was transferred to an adult unit. And really that doesn't happen very often but when things like that do happen, we may hear, 'Why can't you keep these kids under control?' It's that lack of support that hurts. Also there may be conflict with the psychiatrists—sometimes they won't change their approach with the patient even if the approach isn't working.

"In recent years, the period of hospitalization for psychiatric illness has gotten shorter and there's a trend toward more out-patient care. In many cases, however, that's not in the best interest of the patients or their families. We're sending kids home now quicker—but also sicker!"

What does it take to be successful in this specialty? "A good psychiatric nurse has to first be in good physical and emotional shape. She has to be able to differentiate between what's going on in her life and what's going on with the patient. She can't be so judgmental or fixed with certain stereotypes that she can't see the patient as a person. Most important, she has to have compassion for those persons who have emotional problems."

Cathy has been a psychiatric nurse for fifteen years. Prior to obtaining her AD in nursing (through the New York State Regents External Degree Program), she worked in various other nursing specialities but enjoys working with young people in psychiatry the most.

"I'll soon be completing my BSN in preparation for getting my master's in psychiatric nursing. That's important for moving ahead. But most of the skills that I use as a nurse I've learned on the job or through life experiences. My advice to someone considering this field is to read all you can about psychology; to get experience as a counselor, if possible; and to participate in seminars on psychiatry or psychiatric nursing. A nurse has to take responsibility for her own learning and improving her skills—that's being professional."

Liz Fehlberg, a supervisor in a private psychiatric hospital in San Diego, had some additional observations about her specialty:

"The most stressful area to work in psychiatric nursing is the intensive care unit (or, as they were once called, the 'locked wards'). Patients are often out of control, verbally abusive, and require a close watch because of suicidal tendencies. There's high burnout for nurses who work there. Also, the older chronic patients may be difficult because their outlook for improvement is often not good.

"A psychiatric nurse must be capable of performing a wide variety of tasks. She may be called on to start IVs and do tube feedings and catheterizations, so her background in medical-surgical nursing is important. She may also be called on to handle medical emergencies, so experience in the emergency room is also useful.

"The trend in all psychiatric care is for more out-patient treatment. The reason for this is to decrease costs and to increase independence and recovery of patients. This day care is provided through the hospital or a community program and is another area where nurses are providing care."

REHABILITATION NURSING

Tom Lowell, age 22, was in an automobile accident and as a result is paralyzed in both arms and legs (the medical term is *quadriplegia*). At a time in his life when he should be struggling with a career and life decisions, Tom is struggling with his rehabilitation nurse, Carol Bagguley, about starting his day.

"Tom, all patients are expected to get dressed and go to the dining room for breakfast. I know that you can do it too."

"It's too early. I never get up before ten. Why can't you feed me my breakfast—just this once—and then later I'll get up."

"No, Tom. Everyone is getting ready now."

"Well, I'm not. I'm tired."

Besides not wanting to get out of bed, Tom doesn't want to use the strap-on cuff, the splint, and the extended fork that are necessary in order for him to feed himself. He doesn't want to go through the exhausting motions of dressing himself either. Mostly Tom doesn't like his life right now, and he's not thrilled with Ms. Bagguley, who doesn't seem to give up.

"I'll tell you what, Tom. If you get dressed and feed yourself, I'll let you eat in bed. How's that sound?"

It sounds good to Tom. He feels that he's won at least one concession, and Ms. Bagguley, although she had to make a tradeoff, knows that for Tom, working on feeding himself and doing personal care is the important thing now.

Eventually, Tom finds that eating in bed is not as easy as eating in the dining room, and he volunteers to change his morning pattern. He gets out of bed with his three roommates and goes to the dining room for breakfast.

Months later, after intensive work with the members of the rehabilitation team, Tom has started to put his life back in order and not only doesn't fight with Ms. Bagguley any longer but explains to a newly admitted paralyzed patient, "Now listen, friend, you do what these nurses say. In the long run, you'll thank them."

As Tom leaves Sharp Rehabilitation Center, he starts a new life as a disabled person. But his chances for success, both personally and professionally, are greatly enhanced by his three-month experience there. And he will return to the center's outpatient facility to continue all areas of therapy.

Ms. Bagguley explains, "Because of Tom's disability, he was left with very little control over his life. This is a devastating time for him and we're very aware of that. So we made a small tradeoff in the beginning. But we still set the guidelines for his treatment program. A rehabilitation nurse has to be firm, even though the natural tendency is to be soft."

Ms. Bagguley works as a primary nurse on an eight-bed module for patients with spinal cord injuries. This is one section of the fifty-bed rehabilitation center that is a division of Sharp Memorial Hospital in San Diego, California. The center also has 20,272 outpatient visits per year.

Besides the sixteen-bed wing for patients with spinal cord injuries, there are two other wings—one for patients who have strokes and the other for patients with head injuries. There are also facilities for amputees and for persons with other disabilities. Each of the three wings is set apart with its own bright primary color scheme. Some patients' rooms are decorated with lively posters and other personal articles. Instead of carpet on the floors, there's carpet on the walls to protect them from patients who are learning to push their own wheelchairs. The large physical therapy room, the ramps, the lowered sinks, and the sturdy handrails in the halls and in the bathrooms all accommodate the special patients that stay here. There are no patients in traditional hospital garb—they wear their own clothes. The 128 nurses who care for the patients also wear street clothes during working hours.

The rehabilitation team consists of the doctors and nurses as well as physical, occupational, vocational, speech, and recreation therapists. In addition, there are specialists from the fields of social service, psychology, pulmonary care, orthotics, prosthetics, rehab engineering, and nutrition. Representatives from each of these disciplines meet on a regular basis to review patient care and progress.

The nurses coordinate the patients' activities and spend the most time with them during their hospital stay. The nurse's role is not always an easy one. Examination of the patient schedule board indicates the great number of activities in which patients are involved. They move from one therapy to another, and nursing care and teaching are planned around this schedule.

Ideally, patients are admitted to the rehabilitation center as soon as possible after injury or debilitating illness occurs. At this point, the patient is still physically and psychologically vulnerable, so the nurse must be observant for any complications (the usual secondary problems include those affecting the heart, lungs, bowel, skin and bladder). Nursing duties may involve administration of tube feedings, tracheotomy care, catheterizations, bowel and skin care. The psychological depression and shattered self-image is also a factor in nursing care.

"In addition to the role of caregiver, the role of teacher is of primary importance for the rehabilitation nurse," says Aloma (Cookie) Gender, RN, BSN, CRRN, manager of patient care services which includes rehabilitation nursing as well as social services. "The patient and family members must be thoroughly knowledgeable about the patient's illness and be able to take appropriate measures to prevent further complications. In Tom's case, this would include teaching proper skin care and inspection in order to prevent future pressure areas."

Ms. Gender continues, "The rehabilitation nurse must be a generalist as well as a specialist. A knowledge of medical-surgical nursing, critical care, and psychiatric nursing is necessary in caring for the disabled patient as is a specific knowledge of rehabilitation nursing. Since length of stay on a rehabilitation unit is four weeks or longer, the nurse has an opportunity to become acquainted not only with the patient but also with the family. Psychosocial skills are needed to assist both the patient and their significant others to adjust to the disability."

Shirley Santoro has worked as a staff nurse in the unit for patients with head injuries for eight years. In the eight-bed module, there is usually at least another RN or LVN and one aide in addition to Ms. Santoro. Her day begins at seven, although she often arrives earlier in order to evaluate changes with the patients and get the day's activities organized.

"We establish regimens for the patients and set up certain goals. I usually work intensively with three or four patients. Teaching—with patient and family members—is done at the same time that physical care is given and at formal teaching sessions. Staff members are also involved in orienting new personnel.

"Unlike nurses in the acute care setting, the rewards for a rehab nurse come weeks later. A tremendous amount of patience and hopefulness is required when patients have to work against what once were considered insurmountable problems. We're fortunate here that team morale is high—we all pull together. Of course all patients are not success stories. Sometimes the patient's physical injury will not allow him to make gains, and instead of returning home, he must be admitted to a nursing home. But even then, we have the satisfaction of knowing we did the best job we could. And family members have been taught quality nursing care. This can be a great benefit even if the patient is admitted to a nursing home."

At Sharp Rehabilitation Center, there are opportunities for nurses to advance in the clinical setting, as well as administratively, through the career advancement program. Clinical specialists are an important part of the nursing team and continuing education is offered regularly. Carol Bagguley is a Clinical Nurse II and is a graduate of a diploma program. She had previous experience in pediatric and medical-surgical nursing. Shirley Santoro is a Clinical Nurse IV and is also a diploma graduate who spent ten years as a medical nurse before earning her BS degree in health sciences and joining the rehab staff. Both Ms. Bagguley and Ms. Santoro are certified in rehabilitation nursing (CRRN). Examination for certification has been available since 1983 through the Association of Rehabilitation Nurses.

Rehabilitation nursing is growing as a specialty area and the demand for nurses is increasing. Accelerated acute care technology and improved trauma care has increased the number of patients surviving severe illnesses or injuries, and many are left with severe disabilities. The aging population has increased the need for rehab beds, especially in stroke rehabilitation.

Besides working in acute rehab settings, rehabilitation nurses are employed in intensive care units, home health care agencies, community agencies (such as the M.S. Society), skilled nursing facilities, extended care facilities, adult day care and hospices. Outpatient rehab nurses work with physician groups and institutionally based clinics. Insurance rehab nurses work as case managers for disabled clients who have private insurance or worker's compensation injuries. They may be in private practice or work as employees of the insurance company. Rehab nurses in private practice may also serve as expert witnesses or provide lifetime care needs analyses for attorneys in malpractice or civil suits.

Margaret Ford, RN, is employed at Rancho Los Amigos Hospital in Downey, California. One of seven county hospitals in the Los Angeles area, RLAH is the county's only rehabilitation facility and is a regional spinal cord injury center. Ford is a supervising staff nurse on a thirty-bed unit for patients with spinal cord injuries caused by trauma, disease, and birth defects.

Since she works the night shift, her challenges are somewhat different. Ford explains, "This is the only shift in which the patient must interact with just the immediate staff. There are no family, significant others, visitors, students, therapists, or any of the usual constant stream of people that mark his days. Our patients are with us for quite a long time: paraplegics for three to four months and quadriplegics for as long as seven months. So we get to know each other pretty well and this shift can be the first to see signs of conflicts emerging or resolving. The challenge of providing innovative nursing care is never more needed. Ensuring that the patient receives the maximum amount of rest and yet being there when conflicts are present is one of the things I like best about my job. Any able-bodied person can only imagine how a spinal-injured person must feel in the middle of the night with splints, casts, braces, and, of course, pain as constant companions.

"A 'typical' night on my unit, when described, gives the impression of sameness. That's because there are so many seemingly small and trivial tasks that can take up a large percentage of nursing hours. But it is these 'small and trivial' things that make each night different and challenging. For example, finding and relieving a quadriplegic's nagging back itch that has plagued him all day; helping a high paraplegic to cough; adjusting an uncomfortable neck brace so that a good night's sleep can be made possible; helping an emotional young woman tolerate her bulky flexion traction. These are the types of nursing functions that make each tour of duty unique. And I haven't even mentioned any of the life-threatening situations that of course arise from time to time!"

Ford received an AD in nursing in 1978, completed a nine-month spinal-cord-injury nurse practitioner program in 1980 and received a BSN in 1986. She's presently enrolled in an MSN program through the California State University Consortium. Ford received certification in rehabilitation nursing in 1985.

In Ford's view, the most important traits for an effective rehabilitation nurse are patience, tolerance, honesty, and a sense of humor. "In addition, it is important to be able to teach and work as part of a team.

"To any prospective nursing student interested in rehab nursing, I would point out several things. First, she should be aware of the demand that nursing in general will make and then consider that rehab nursing will probably double these demands. Secondly, I would suggest that she take a personal inventory in terms of the qualities I have cited. She should examine her gut feeling about the long-term disabled patient who requires total care. She should get in touch with how she handles loss, how she deals with failures. And of course, I would point out the rewards and the deep sense of satisfaction she can attain from this type of nursing."

Other Rehabilitation Units

Nurses may also be employed in alcoholic or drug rehab units, where patients receive specialized care while withdrawing from alcohol or drug abuse. Usually these are part of an acute hospital but can be a separate institution. Nurses are part of the team that works with these patients, and their families, in returning the addict to a healthier life-style.

Cardiac rehab units usually function as satellites of hospitals. Nurses teach heart patients proper diet and other facts concerning normal and abnormal heart function. In addition, areas are set aside in or near the hospitals where a number of recuperating heart patients exercise in a group. The nurse has monitoring and crash cart equipment at the ready as she directs the patients in their exercise routines. A nurse working in this setting usually has a strong background in medicine and surgery.

There are also opportunities for rehab nurses in the subspecialties of arthritis, cancer, diabetes, degenerative neurological diseases and other areas. Whether practicing in a large specialized center or as part of a general hospital structure, the rehabilitation nurse helps the handicapped person to return to the mainstream of society and be as independent as possible.

NURSING HOMES

Geriatrics (the branch of medicine that deals with the diseases and problems of the elderly) is a rapidly growing field and many nurses practice this specialty in nursing homes. Nursing homes are found all across the country but are particularly popular in the sunbelt states. In this area, there is a shortage of geriatric nurses and many facilities use agency nurses to fill out their licensed staff.

Karen Malik is an LVN who has worked in many southern California nursing homes, both part-time and full-time. For a number of years, she's worked through a nursing agency and rotates among four homes in the San Diego area. Nurse Malik explains her feelings about working in these facilities:

"There are all kinds of nursing homes. Some are well run, but many are managed poorly and operate on such low budgets that food is poor and supplies are scarce. Lack of bed linen is a constant problem. And when you have to count disposable rubber gloves at the end of a shift, you know something's very wrong. Even in the best of nursing homes,

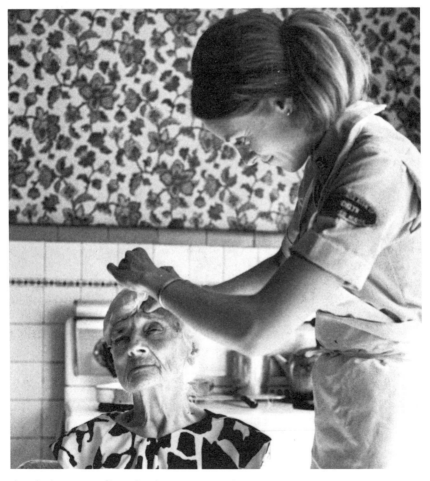

A geriatric nurse applies a dressing to a patient. *(Courtesy Scripps Memorial Hospital)*

licensed personnel are in short supply, and because aides are paid only the minimum wage, many of them have limited education, are unreliable, and may be abusive to the patients. The work is not glamorous and is physically hard. You have to turn and lift patients and you're on your feet a lot.

"The real problem with nursing homes is that older people are often stripped of their privacy, dignity, and their will to live. Many times family members abandon them. It can be sad.

"But after having said all that, I must add that some of the most dedicated and creative nurses I've known work in nursing homes. The facility is their second home and they consider the patients 'family.' Many practical nurses find work in nursing homes satisfying because they have a higher level of authority, responsibility, and independence in a nursing home than in an acute-care hospital. Also, this is a field where nurses are able to build long-term relationships with the patients and their families. And that can be very satisfying.

"Eight years ago, for example, I worked in a home in Anaheim and cared for a woman patient for several years. Her husband would visit every day and we became good friends. I tried to make things as comfortable as I could for Mrs. Kingston, but after three years, she died. That was five years ago but I still keep in touch with Mr. Kingston. He sort of adopted me and vice versa."

Nurse Malik usually works the evening shift and is responsible for passing medications, giving treatments, and carrying out doctors' orders for fifty patients. In a one-hundred-bed facility (the usual size in the San Diego area), she works with another LVN, who is responsible for the other fifty patients.

Arriving at the home at 3:00, Malik takes report from the day nurse and then sets up her medications and passes them out between 4:00 and 5:00. This period may be interrupted by doctors' calls as orders are changed. At 6:00 there's a supper break, then time for charting and other paperwork. Evening medications are given at 8:00 or 9:00, and then treatments are done. This may include care of bedsores, colostomy care, dressing changes—whatever is necessary. The evening shift is over at 11:00, after the report is given to the night nurse.

"I think a nurse's worst fear is that a patient will die on her shift, and you see a lot of death in the nursing home. Usually it's not a sad occasion, because the patients want to die. I remember one conversation very vividly. Mrs. Allen was a favorite of mine. One evening I was treating her bed sore and getting her ready for bed. She said, 'I just wish I could go to sleep and the Lord would take me.' My immediate impulse was to say, 'Oh now you don't mean that.' But Mrs. Allen seemed very comfortable with the thought of dying. I was the one that wasn't comfortable. So I said, 'You really do feel this way, don't you?' She explained that she was old and blind and had to depend on other people—a situation she didn't like—and, all things considered, she was ready to go.

"We talked for quite a while that evening. Mrs. Allen was very matter-of-fact. She wasn't feeling great self-pity but just felt that life was now a burden and she wanted out. Afterwards, I thought, 'What a peace that must be to feel that way.'

"I have, of course, gotten emotionally involved with patients—every nurse does that at one time or another. One evening I was passing medications and was helping Mrs. Angelini back to bed. She was a dear person and I often pampered her if I had the time. I'd get her a drink of water and tuck the blankets in around her. As I was doing this, she looked up at me and said, 'You are so kind to me. Let me kiss you.' I bent over and she kissed my cheek. It touched me so much that I could barely get out of the room before giving in to tears. I felt that I was able to do so little for this dear lady and I felt guilty that I wouldn't be there every night to tuck her in."

It's been estimated that one-fourth of patients in nursing homes do not need to be there. With a little help from outside services, they could remain at home—a much better alternative—for a little longer. Both public and private health care agencies can provide extra health care and housekeeping services that can mean the difference between independence and institutional care. And in many states, there are day care centers for the elderly. Staffed by nurses, physical therapists, and nutritionists, these centers monitor older handicapped patients and provide them with needed medical services. Patients usually spend two to three days a week (from 10:00 a.m. to 3:00 p.m.) at these centers, receive health supervision, participate in an exercise and social program, and receive a nourishing meal. The remainder of their time is spend at home. These day care centers should not be confused with senior citizens' centers, which are not equipped to care for the handicapped person.

Nurses working in these areas function as coordinators, practitioners, and therapists. Their responsibilities vary according to the center's size and function and the population it serves.

Day care centers are of course not the answer for every older infirm person, but they do provide dignity and independence for many. And a big advantage is that they cost much less than nursing home care.

IN THE COMMUNITY

Are you interested in spending your summers working with adventurous children in the out-of-doors? Then you might consider a job in camp nursing.

Would you find working in an infirmary or health office in a state prison to be a challenging and worthwhile experience? Many nurses do.

Some nurses find that a career in pharmaceutical sales is the way to go. This field, although limited to the baccalaureate graduate, provides an independent workstyle as the nurse travels from one client to the next promoting the products she represents.

Utilization review nurses (see Chapter 6) now find opportunities for employment not only in hospitals but also in insurance companies and various health agencies.

Opportunities abound for nursing outside the hospital. Besides employment in the traditional areas of physicians' offices, public health, school health, and occupational health, there are some new specialty areas in which nurses are becoming involved.

One is the area of self-care, in which community nurses encourage their patients to take more responsibility for their health and teach them certain skills that are useful in determining when and if medical care is needed.

Backing up even a step further are the health promotion and education centers, where the emphasis is on preventing disease by focusing on the patient's life-style and motivating clients to change unhealthy living patterns.

One such center, called The Well Being, is located in a shopping center in La Jolla, California. As an outreach of Scripps Memorial Hospitals Foundation, the center has four components: (1) a classroom area where instructors or hospital staff nurses teach classes on childbirth preparation, diet, exercise, and other areas of health promotion; (2) a consumer-oriented library stocked with books, pamphlets, and audio-visual materials; (3) a display center sponsored in conjunction with local health agencies (the health theme display changes every three months); and (4) a referral service where health problems are evaluated and the client is referred to the proper community source.

Kim Moreno, RN, is the Director of this center and works autonomously as an outreach of the hospital. She feels that the area of health promotion is a natural for nurses in that their communication skills and knowledge of the behavioral sciences are brought into play.

"The best part of my job is the constant challenge of trying to find what will motivate people to change. There's also the excitement of working with many groups in the community and getting involved in the public relations part of health promotion. I'm frequently asked, for example, to speak at community groups or am being interviewed by newspaper reporters. Health promotion is a growing area—the medical community as well as the public needs to be educated on what we can do. We feel that health is not only the absence of disease but is the observance of such positive habits as exercise, proper diet, nonsmoking, and stress management. These are some of the areas that we are involved in here. The center has an advisory board made up of health professionals and community leaders—they help us in making policy decisions. There's one other full-time nurse on staff."

Director Moreno has an MS and many years of nursing experience. For the nurse considering a career in health promotion, communication skills are very important. To become a director, for whom decision-making and knowledge of the business world are necessary, it's useful to have some experience in marketing, negotiating, and accounting. The Well Being center is presently funded by private grant money and charges for some services. "Eventually we hope to be self-supporting, and that's why the business skills are so important."

Kim Moreno enjoys an excellent salary as Director of the center and has been involved in the program from the time it was just an idea. The Well Being, one of a growing number of storefront health-education facilities across the nation, represents a new health care plan: providing alternative ways for people to maintain and improve their health.

Office Nurse

Outside the hospital, many people connect the role of nurse with the white-uniformed woman who performs the clerical and some of the medical-assistant tasks of a busy doctor's office. This person, however, isn't necessarily either an LVN/LPN or an RN. Many medical assistants are trained in short vocational programs or receive training on the job from the physician. Some nurses, of course, do work in doctors' offices and some work in the expanded role of nurse practitioner. The nurse practitioner examines, diagnoses, and treats certain patients with the physician acting as supervisor. These nurses will be followed more closely in Chapter 9.

A new type of office nurse has recently appeared—she is a member of a team that works at urgent or immediate care clinics. These facilities—a cross between a hospital emergency room and a family doctor's office—are usually privately owned and offer reduced cost walk-in care for minor emergencies and medical problems. Because of their lower cost, greater convenience and more personalized service, urgent care clinics have become very popular across the country.

Doctors Care Medical Centers has three urgent care facilities located in the southern California cities of Escondido, Carlsbad, and Oceanside. These facilities, open seven days a week, twelve hours a day, are doctor owned and operated and staff a primary care physician, an emergency nurse, an X-ray technician, a lab technician and a secretary/receptionist.

Barbara Saad, RN is the nursing manager of these urgent care centers. She explains the nurse's duties: "Since there is usually only one nurse on duty at a time, she has a great deal of responsibility. It's for this reason that we hire nurses who have had previous hospital experience in the areas of emergency room or critical care. The nurse acts as a triage person to determine who needs care first. For example, if a patient has severe pain (especially in the chest), severe bleeding or chemical burns in the eye, that patient will be seen immediately. If the problem is serious, the patient will be stabilized at our center then sent by ambulance to the local hospital.

"Once inside the examination area, the nurse takes the patient's history, does a brief examination including vital signs and asks questions to help focus the chief complaint. The nurse anticipates tests or procedures that may be necessary and sets up the needed equipment or supplies.

"Perhaps the most important aspect of our care is caring. If a patient feels uncomfortable enough to seek medical attention, it's not a trivial matter. A bothersome cold may not be as dramatic as a high speed freeway accident, but our patients are more aware of their surroundings and the attitudes of their caregivers. They know the potential consequences and threats to their well-being that a somewhat minor problem can cause. We understand and respect the patient's fears and try to do everything possible to make the total experience a pleasant one. We teach when questions arise and offer suggestions (besides medication) to shorten recovery times.

"We also give health guidance by telephone either directing home first aid or helping patients decide when it's appropriate to be re-examined. Other duties of an urgent care nurse include: cleaning wounds, applying dressings and splints, performing certain tests, giving medications and immunizations, as well as restocking supplies and sterilizing instruments.

Ms. Saad, like many other nurses in her position, had considerable nursing experience before becoming nursing manager. She received her RN through an AA degree program then later received a BS degree in Nursing Science and is looking forward to beginning an MBA program. Nurse Saad was an emergency room staff nurse for thirteen years with over four years of charge responsibilities in the emergency room. She was certified as a mobile intensive care nurse (MICN) and taught classes to emergency medical technicians.

In her present position as nursing manager, much of Nurse Saad's time is spent in interviewing and hiring personnel, supervising staff members, ordering supplies, problem solving, and writing up policy and procedure manuals as well as writing aftercare instruction sheets for patients. She also stays active in her professional organizations (Occupational Health Nurses Association and Emergency Nurses Association).

"Working as an urgent care nurse offers many challenges. As the nurse tries to meet patients' needs, she also has the creative challenge of putting programs together. Because this is such a new field, there are many opportunities to set standards and determine policies. In this type of setting, a nurse can learn a great deal about private business, marketing, public relations and customer satisfaction while still maintaining patient contact."

Nurse Saad is honest in pointing out some of the disadvantages in this field of nursing, "Salary and benefits are usually less than nurses in the hospital receive although salaries are better than nurses who work in traditional doctor's offices. And there's always more work to do than you can get done. But that's a common problem in nursing!"

What kind of person makes a good urgent care nurse? Ms. Saad explains, "The nurse is a key person in coordinating office activities. For that reason, she needs to be well-organized yet flexible. An urgent care nurse must be secure about herself and her skills so this is not usually a good job for a nurse just out of school. Experience in emergency room or critical care nursing is probably best. Most importantly, a nurse in this field must really like people and be able to offer acceptance and reassurance to patients and staff."

In addition to urgent care clinics, nurses may be employed in surgical day care centers or "surgicenters." As a response to increased costs and impersonal hospital care, such minor surgical procedures as tonsillectomies, simple eye or cosmetic surgery, tissue biopsies, and abortions may now be done on an outpatient basis. Surgical centers are either privately owned or are satellites of large hospitals. Patients arrive early in the morning at the centers, have surgery, then recover for several hours before returning home. Nurses working in these

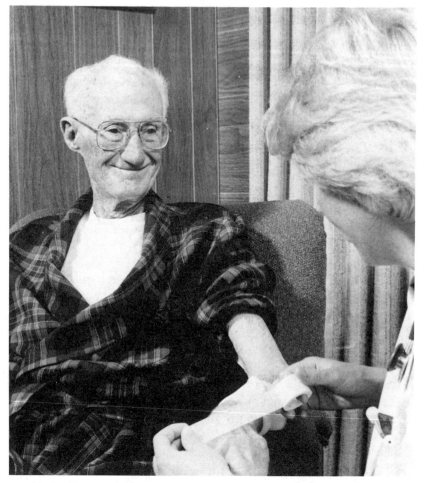

A public health nurse examines a patient in the patient's home. *(Photo by Sandra Weiner)*

areas have a background in surgical nursing and work in much the same capacity as their hospital counterparts. This includes preoperative patient teaching and support. After surgery, nurses monitor patients' vital signs and check dressings, drainage, IV infusions, and circulation. Nurses also arrange with the patients and their families for care at home and for a follow-up office visit with the surgeon.

Home Health Nurse

For four years, Donnette M. Ohlsson ("Dee") has been a public health nurse at Allied Home Health Association in San Diego. For the last year, she's been the admission's nurse which means she visits newly referred patients and decides, after consulting with the doctor, what nursing care the agency will provide.

One summer afternoon, Nurse Ohlsson is preparing to make her fourth visit of the day (this is the usual number for an admission's nurse although other staff nurses typically make five to six visits per day).

After completing paper work at her desk, Nurse Ohlsson puts on a short white lab coat over her regular clothes and grabs her briefcase which holds charts and records. The southern California sun is momentarily blinding as she walks to her parked car.

The patient that she will visit next lives about 10 miles from the office so, before starting her car, the nurse examines a detailed map to figure out the best way to get to the patient's house.

"A map is an important piece of equipment for a home health nurse. You don't want to spend anymore time than you have to in travel."

Although Ohlsson would literally be lost without her map, it's by no means the only equipment she carries with her. "I pretty much live out of my car," explains the blond-haired Ohlsson with a twinkle in her eye. "I carry a cooler filled with food and I have other personal items as well as patients' records and office paper work. Then I have two basic equipment bags. One I carry to almost all visits since I do physical assessments. This bag includes a stethoscope, blood pressure cuff, thermometer, otoscope (to examine ears), 'sticks' for testing urine, small dressings and examining gloves. My other equipment bag is specifically for blood work—taking specimens, starting IVs. And the trunk of my car is filled with various supplies. Maybe I carry too much but it's terrible to get out in the field and not have what I need. We often use the latest equipment and newest techniques with our patients." Ohlsson explains, "What works in the hospital isn't always what works best at home. More and more, we're getting complicated cases that require a lot of creativity to provide the best possible care."

"This morning, for example, I visited two very ill patients who will require frequent visits by the staff nurse. The first, a 50-year-old woman, is very overweight and has serious circulatory problems that resulted in amputation of one leg and contributed to three draining wounds (one wound is on the leg stump and another is on the hip— the third occurred after abdominal surgery). All of these wounds are serious and require the professional care of a nurse."

Ohlsson continues, "Because the patient is so large and no longer has bowel or bladder control, she needs two people to move her and assist in her daily care. So besides nursing visits, the home health aide will be providing personal care and chore services. Fortunately, the woman's husband is at home and is very helpful. This patient is in a hospital bed and frankly, a few years back, she would have received care in the hospital rather than at home.

"The other patient that I saw this morning was a 26-year-old single man who was just released after a two week stay in the hospital. He has a serious bone infection on his hand and will require five visits today, two visits tomorrow, then a visit every day for three days with visits gradually tapering off after that." Why so many visits? "This man is receiving antibiotics through an IV (intravenous) solution and that requires close monitoring. In addition to the IV treatment, he'll need frequent wound care for the hand. Besides that, we'll monitor his progress with blood tests (for which we draw the blood and deliver the specimen to the lab) and will keep in close touch with the physician in charge."

Nurse Ohlsson pauses for a moment and explains, "Many patients are now sent home from the hospital earlier (and sicker), the home health nurse often performs complex, highly technical nursing tasks such as instituting and supervising IV therapy, monitoring treatment with ventilators, oxygen, or suction equipment. In fact, the list of nursing care that can be provided at home is quite long. The challenges for today's home health nurse have never been greater!"

A half hour after leaving the office, Ohlsson finds a parking place in front of a modest one family home. This is her fourth visit of the day and the nurse examines her referral notes, "Mr. Campbell is a 91-year-old widower who just got out of the hospital following five weeks' treatment for a stroke. He belongs to an HMO and they'll be sending out a physical therapist and an occupational therapist to work with him. The HMO nurse was too busy to come and asked if I would make an evaluation visit to see how he's getting along. There may be a need for help with diet and medication."

Because Ms. Ohlsson has called ahead, Mr. Campbell is waiting for her. He sits on the couch in his living room watching television. When the nurse enters, he turns off the television with a remote, control device and greets the nurse with a warm smile. Neatly dressed in slacks, shirt and sneakers, the only evidence of "disability" is the aluminum cane that rests beside him and a walker that can be seen in the next room. Although slightly hard of hearing, the retired salesman answers all the nurse's questions concerning his illness and social situation.

"Can you tell me what happened to you that you had to go to the hospital?"

"I fell over and Mike—that's my grandson—picked me up and took me in. I had a stroke."

As the nurse asks the necessary questions and Mr. Campbell answers them, Ohlsson fills out the agency's "problem-plan list" that determines the nursing diagnosis for all home care patients. With Mr. Campbell, for example, Ohlsson finds out that medication and diet are not really a problem and, in fact, the elderly gentleman is managing quite well.

Campbell explains, "Before Mike goes to work in the morning, he makes me a thermos of coffee and some sandwiches. That gets me by 'till he comes home at three o'clock."

The nurse pauses for a moment then comments, "It sounds like your grandson cares for you. You're fortunate and he's fortunate." The elderly man smiles.

Having asked all her questions, Nurse Ohlsson washes her hands and does a physical assessment. She takes Mr. Campbell's temperature, blood pressure, pulse, and listens to his heart and lungs. The nurse reports her findings, "Your blood pressure is 142 over 80 and that's okay for your age." With a trained eye, she examines the man's skin, checks for swelling in the ankles and evaluates the degree of weakness in the arm that was affected by the stroke. Ohlsson watches her patient walk and concludes, "I don't think you need a nurse, Mr. Campbell, but you do need physical therapy. The therapist should help you particularly with getting in and out of the car and the bathtub—even though you use a stool for your shower."

The visit concludes with the nurse's invitation to, "Call if you need help—I'm leaving one of our brochures with you."

After returning to her car, Ohlsson explains, "This is not a complicated case and there'll be no need for me to visit again unless Mr. Campbell's condition changes. Usually, after making an assessment visit, I would go back to the office and speak to the doctor in charge and tell him (or her) my recommended treatment plan. There are very few doctors that don't agree with our recommendations. Then, after getting a verbal okay, we receive written approval and the treatment program begins."

Allied Home Health Association has been in business for 16 years and serves the entire San Diego county out of two offices. There are 25 nurses on staff and the majority are public health nurses (this means the nurses have completed an NLN approved baccalaureate program and have been certified by the state). There's also one nurse practitioner and 45 contract nurses who work on a fee for service basis. In addition, there are 18 home health aides and two social workers on staff as well as additional contract social workers and contract physical, occupational and speech therapists. Staff nurses manage their own geographic area and are assigned patients after Nurse Ohlsson makes the evaluation visits and receives approval from the physician and the third party provider. Most nurses are assigned to the 8 a.m. to 5 p.m. shift although some work from 2 p.m. to 10:30 p.m. In addition, there's one nurse on call from 10:30 p.m. until 8 a.m.

One of the most unique aspects of the role of today's home health nurse is that of professional assessor. As an admission's nurse, Dee Ohlsson's asssignments typify the complex task of working with many different disciplines and using many different skills.

The path that Dee Ohlsson followed to become a public health nurse is somewhat different than the usual nurse. She worked as a bookkeeper in a department store until age 32 when she decided to go back to school. "I decided to go into nursing not because I had to but because I wanted to. I first got my AA degree then received my baccalaureate from Arizona State University at Tempe. I also have 16 hours toward my Master's degree." Before joining the San Diego agency, Ohlsson worked for five years as charge nurse in the respiratory unit of an Arizona geriatric hospital. "There were many reasons why I decided to go into home health nursing but one big plus that immediately comes to mind is the regular Monday through Friday daytime schedule that we enjoy. Working every fifth or sixth week-end is not that much of an inconvenience. And then too I enjoy the independence that goes along with the job."

Suzanne Wunsch is Associate Director of Patient Services at Allied Home Health Association. When asked what she looks for in a home health nurse, the director was very explicit, "We want a baccalaureate nurse with five years experience in public health or acute care nursing. Some clinical specialists have MS degrees. Occasionally we may hire a diploma graduate with special technical skills. Besides educational criteria, I look for a mature nurse who understands the nursing process thoroughly and enjoys working with people of all ages. Technical skills are important and, whether we like it or not, so are writing skills since clear, concise paperwork is now such an important part of the job."

As many health specialists are quick to point out, the role of the home health nurse has changed considerably over the years. Until recently, home health care was provided mostly by visiting nurses or public health nurses. The RN who worked for a visiting nurse association (hence the name visiting nurse) often gave routine nursing care and provided health guidance in the home. The agency charged for these services. The public health nurse (an RN with a minimum baccalaureate degree as well as official certification) worked in a health department setting and coordinated services to improve the health and well-being of the community. The public health nurse also made home visits to provide health guidance and limited physical care. Until recently, these services were free.

Today, there are new providers in the home health care field and the job of the home health nurse has changed radically. Besides visiting nurse associations and health departments, home health care can be provided by hospital-based agencies, proprietary (profit-making) agencies and private, nonprofit agencies (Allied Home Health Association fits in this category).

Pam Hardiman, director of health services at the Tampa Visiting Nurses' Association (VNA) in Tampa, Florida, explains the qualities that she looks for in a visiting nurse: "Doctors often write orders that say, 'Evaluate and treat.' The nurse must develop an acceptable care plan and treatment based on *her* observations and judgment. She must, therefore, have a good background in medical-surgical nursing, be self-assured and even assertive. She should be organized yet flexible and should like being independent. Being a visiting nurse puts to work all those skills that nurses learn in school but are not able to use in other jobs.

"If a high school student is interested in home nursing care, she should contact her local home health agency, VNA, or health department and go out with one of the nurses for a day. We do that here."

Although health departments are no longer the most common employer of public health nurses, many still hire nurses to provide home care as well as other health services. Health departments may also employ physicians, environmental engineers, statisticians, health educators and other personnel to carry out various programs.

Liz Macris is a public health nurse in the Rensselaer County Health Department in upstate New York. Besides making home visits, Nurse Macris works once a month in the tuberculosis and chest clinic where she interviews patients, collects specimens, dispenses medication, and works with the clinic doctor in giving follow-up care. Less often, Macris works in the venereal disease clinic, and her responsibilities there are much the same as in the chest clinic. She does not work in the immunization clinics (RNs supervise these) but does work fairly often (between one and three times per month) in the well-baby clinic.

"There's no other nursing job where you can be on your own as much as you are in public health," says Nurse Macris. "Usually I plan my own day and use my own judgment, while still working under doctor's orders. What really makes the job is that patients rely on the home health nurse for support and they see her in a professional role.

The other side of the coin, of course, is that dealing with patients and meeting the needs of the whole family can be emotionally draining. In the hospital, the nurse's concern is usually only with the patient. In home health care, there's the rest of the family plus the social and economic conditions in which patients live. The nurse is often exposed to lice, roaches, rats, garbage, and unclean homes. Then there's the traveling in all kinds of weather. That's all part of the job.

"A good home health nurse is sensitive, caring, and kind. She should like working with people, be aware of their needs, and have a desire to care for the sick and disabled. At the same time, there are limitations to what one person can do, and help must be sought when necessary. A home health nurse must be a good listener and observer and should be able to work with other people well. This includes patients, co-workers, and superiors."

School Nurse

Most adults picture a school nurse as the person who provides first aid for sickness and accidents during school hours (although the nurse is not allowed to give even an aspirin to a student). They also may think of the school nurse as the one who keeps records and does the eye and ear screening exams. Maybe there's some health teaching too. But mostly the job is pretty dull, right? Don't count on it!

Chances are that someone who is hired to do just those tasks is not a nurse at all but a health aide. The real nurse is more likely to act in a consultant role or, in the best of all worlds, she's a nurse practitioner who's making a dynamic difference in health care for today's school children.

Sue Carson-Leonard, RN, school nurse practitioner, is the Executive Director of an innovative program in the Denver, Colorado area. There are three other nurse practitioners who serve the high school, two middle schools, and eight elementary schools in the school district. Carson-Leonard explains how the program, called Commerce City Community Health Services, works. "There are full-time health clerks in each school who provide first aid to the students. Then there are three school nurses who rotate between the schools and do the screening exams and some health guidance. Each of the three nurse practitioners is responsible for a certain number of schools and provides care to the students in a clinic-like setting in that school. We have a physician who acts as consultant and spends two half-days per week at the school. For the most part, the nurse practitioners work independently and do physical examinations, assessments, and prescribe a therapeutic program, working under a prescribed medical protocol. We also provide consultation and care for severely and profoundly developmentally delayed children. The job is an exciting one!"

A typical day for one of the nurse practitioners might run like this: "We meet at 8:00 a.m. at our main office in one of the schools. It is here that we examine throat cultures (we also do some other simple screening tests, although the more complex ones are sent out to a private laboratory). If there are any positive throat cultures, we call the parents and the pharmacist. We may contact parents for other follow-up, or they may call us seeking health guidance. Since we provide a twenty-four-hour-per-day telephone consultation service for parents, there may need to be follow-up on calls that came in the night before. There may be referrals to and from other agencies and other reports that need to be written. By 9:00, this work should be completed. We then grab our equipment (instruments, supplies, and books) and start out to the schools. None of the nurses wear traditional uniforms.

"We schedule certain days to visit specific schools, but often there's a problem at another school, so between 9:00 and 10:30 we may go to one of those schools to see sick children, evaluate their problems, and plan a treatment program or provide health guidance. From 10:30 until 2:00, we try to be at the school where we're scheduled for the day. This work may involve follow-up on ear or lung infections or continuing guidance on acne or stress-related problems. We also do routine physical examinations for students, including those in sports programs.

"Late in the afternoon we may be back at another school seeing some students who got sick during the day. By 3:30, we return to the main office and do our lab work or get specimens ready to be sent off to the private laboratory. There may also be a meeting with the Community Advisory Board or some other organizational business."

The school health program, which began in November 1979 (Carson-Leonard joined the group in September 1980 and became Director in 1986) is funded by grants from private foundations and donations from individuals, businesses and community organizations. The program also receives insurance payments for primary care services and charges a yearly membership fee of $40 per child. The program now serves 1,200 children. "If a child is sick at school but is not a member of the program, the service is explained and made available to the family," says Director Carson-Leonard. "The parent can then either accept or reject the services of the nurse."

In analyzing what qualities are important for a nurse in this position, Carson-Leonard explains that "being sensitive to others and being able to get along with many different people—students, parents, faculty, community leaders—are probably most important. We function without much formal structure and work on our own most of the time. One of the school nurse practitioners acts as supervisor, and she relates to the director of student health services. We all are responsible to the School Health Corporation Board.

"It's important to have good clinical skills in this position, and we soon learn that the unexpected should always be expected. There are many interruptions during the day, and sometimes we have to alternate between doing our nursing jobs and doing the organizational things that are required to keep the program going.

"Some of the other pressures are that there's never enough time, and the nurse may be tempted to hurry or not be thorough when she knows other people are waiting. Or we may make people unhappy when we follow proper medical protocol that contradicts a parent's expectations—prescribing penicillin is a good example of this.

"But the job is never boring, and the work we do with the students and parents is usually very gratifying. There was one high school boy who, like the rest of his family, suffered from high blood pressure. He was convinced he was going to die and had essentially given up on himself. He was evaluated and a treatment program was begun. We got his blood pressure down so that he could see some hope for his life. The boy worked on other personal changes and now has a much more positive attitude about his future.

"Another high school student, a girl, had diabetes since the age of nine. For seven years she resisted learning about her disease. Then she came to us, and with an adult acceptance of her condition and of herself, she learned all that she had missed during those years. It was a pleasure to help her because the motivation was there.

"Sometimes more work needs to be done with the parents than with the child. Maybe a parent can't accept a handicap that's holding the student back, or maybe they can't see that their behavior is too controlling. Trying to keep their child in a dependent state is unhealthy for everyone.

"One high school girl came to us and on her third visit said, 'I need to see a psychiatrist!' It seemed she had been sexually abused for six years and finally wanted to get out of the situation. It's a privilege to be able to help someone like that.

"Of course most of our work is not as dramatic as this. We help students find ways to change their life-styles and to improve their health by proper nutrition, exercise, and better self-awareness. We don't always see changes right away, but we hope that somewhere down the road we've made a difference."

Sue Carson-Leonard is a diploma graduate who later obtained her BSN and completed the school nurse practitioner program at the University of Colorado (some school nurses who function in the expanded role have master's degrees, and some are trained as pediatric nurse practitioners). Carson-Leonard's work experiences before she became a school nurse were in the areas of medical, psychiatric, and public health nursing.

For others considering a career in this field, Carson-Leonard suggests volunteering in a school health room. "Spend some time with it. Pay attention to who you are and what you like. Make sure you understand the political structure and the restraints that will be placed on you before taking a position."

Sue Carson-Leonard has worked in school nursing since 1974. But her present position, with its increased independence and responsibility, is "the best." Job satisfaction, for her, is very high. And this has made all the difference in the world.

Occupational Health Nurse

Esther Clauson, RN, sits at her desk in her office filling out medical forms. The door opens and a young man walks in: "Esther, I cut my hand again."

The nurse calmly gets up from her seat and moves toward the young maintenance worker. "What happened Bob?"

"I cut my hand on a piece of sheet metal—went right through the glove—my supervisor said I should come in and show it to ya."

Nurse Clauson examines the hand. "This one doesn't look so bad. Not like some you've had. Let's scrub it up and get you bandaged."

Nurse Clauson knows Bob Vincent pretty well and carries on a friendly conversation with him as she treats his cut. She has a warm smile and a relaxed, easy manner. Her uniform is casual—white pants and shoes, and a pink sweater over a white blouse. An average of twenty-five workers come to the health office every day. With a standing order from the company doctor, she dispenses decongestants for runny noses, throat lozenges for sore throats, and antacids for upset stomachs. She applies hot packs for sprains and reinforces dressings. She gives health advice and listens to people's troubles. Esther Clauson, an occupational health nurse at a manufacturing company in El Cajon, California, explains her work:

"This kind of job isn't for everyone. Each workplace is different, and that makes the nursing job different too. I'm fortunate, from a legal and medical point of view, to have a medical director who supervises much of the program. He's an occupational health doctor for two other industrial companies, and even though he's only here five hours a week, I can always get in touch with him if it's necessary. In our work environment, there's always potential for major accidents. This plant, which employs over a 1,000 people, makes electronic equipment, aerospace hardware, and nuclear piping. I have to be prepared at all times for serious injuries. We've had two partial finger amputations since I've been here and also a serious head injury. In these cases, I gave immediate emergency care, contacted the company doctor, and then arranged for the patient and the appropriate doctor to meet at the hospital."

In addition to emergency care, the medical department is required to do physical examinations of each new employee as well as examinations of employees who return to work after an illness, whether the illness was work related or not. Nurse Clauson's responsibility in these assessments is to take a brief history and do hearing, vision, and urinalysis exams. She also keeps up with the necessary paperwork. Each new employee receives individual counseling from the nurse on safety rules and policies. In addition, if there is a serious plant accident, Nurse Clauson and the chairman of the safety department investigate the incident together.

Twice a year, the medical department sponsors a bloodmobile, and in the summer months, company members are trained or recertified in first aid and CPR techniques. Nurse Clauson is heavily involved in these programs, but as she goes on to explain, "a great amount of my work here is in the nature of counseling. I don't hire or fire, so employees know they can come to me with their troubles. They know I'll listen and I care, and most important, they know that information will never go any further than this office. We have some employees here with serious medical problems. I sometimes have to be the one to evaluate their ability to do the job, or I may be the one to whom they pour out their troubles."

Esther Clauson has been an occupational health nurse for 13 years. Before that, she worked for five years as an emergency room nurse and spent eight years working part-time in pediatrics, obstetrics, and orthopedic nursing. She is a diploma graduate and has been certified as an occupational health nurse for over five years. The criteria for taking the certification examination is that the candidate has to have been in a full-time occupational health position for a minimum of five years. Additional coursework is also required. Clauson is active in the local occupational health nurse organization and finds it gratifying that the membership is continually growing.

Occupational health is not a new specialty, but interest in it has been increasing in recent years. Beginning in the late 1800s, in industries and then in department stores, employers recognized the economic value of keeping their employees healthy, so they began hiring nurses to work on the premises. In 1911, workmen's compensation laws were enacted, and since employers now had to accept responsibility for on-the-job accidents, they saw even more need for safety and first aid programs. Until 1958, nurses in this specialty were known as industrial nurses. Besides working in industrial areas, occupational health nurses are employed in department stores, hotels, and offices. In larger organizations, the nurse works under a medical director. In a smaller company, the nurse may be accountable to management and takes total responsibility for her program.

An occupational health nurse must know about worker's compensation laws and have knowledge of community services. The nurse may have to write reports and be aware of business practices. There may be great emphasis on health education, in which case the nurse may edit bulletins and newsletters.

Nurses in occupational health enjoy good working hours and conditions. Their salary and level of responsibility varies with each employer; some nurses have a great deal of independence and flexibility. Occupational health may not be challenging enough for some nurses—the physical care given is usually routine, and there is not the excitement and stimulation that can be found in hospital nursing. The patient population stays relatively stable—this has both advantages and disadvantages.

Nurse Clauson explains, "More and more, I see jobs opening up in this area. We've proved our worth, and companies are anxious to provide proper medical services for their employees."

AROUND THE WORLD

No matter where a nurse goes in this world, there's a need for her services. It isn't surprising then that many nurses have combined professional skills with a life-style of travel and adventure. Such agencies as the World Health Organization (WHO) and the State

Department offer a limited number of positions in foreign posts. And some nurses strike out on their own to work in overseas hospitals or for private industries. Such positions can be financially rewarding and, at the same time, allow the nurse to experience life in a foreign land. What are some other ways that nurses can practice their profession while they "see the world?"

Military Nursing

ARMY.   For the baccalaureate nursing graduate, the Army provides opportunities in clinical nursing, research and development, and administration. There are nine nursing specialties, including medical-surgical, pediatrics, and community health. An Army nurse may apply for clinical specialty courses, such as intensive care, operating room nursing, community health and environmental science, psychiatric-mental health nursing, anesthesia nursing, pediatrics, adult medical-surgical health care, or obstetrics and gynecology. A nurse-midwifery course and a nursing anesthesia course are also available. In addition, an Army nurse can apply to attend a graduate degree program as a duty assignment. If selected, he or she receives tuition, pay, and allowances

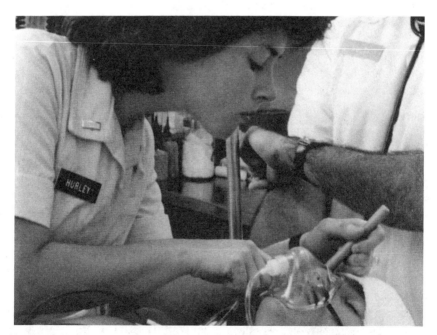

An attending Army nurse checks neurological signs of a patient. *(Courtesy U.S. Army Recruiting Command)*

while attending a civilian university full-time. It should be noted, however, that most advanced specialty courses and degree programs incur an additional service obligation.

In order to qualify for a commission in the Army Nurse Corps, a nurse must meet the following criteria:

1. Have graduated from a baccalaureate school of nursing acceptable to the Department of the Army and accredited by an agency recognized by the United States Secretary of Education.

2. Be at least 21 years of age.

3. Possess a current license to practice nursing in any state of the United States or District of Columbia, or be eligible to take the licensing examination.

4. Be a citizen of the United States (or lawfully admitted to the United States for permanent residence).

5. Meet moral and physical standards prescribed for appointment in the United States Army.

6. Be able to provide professional references.

An Army nurse is a member of a health care system that includes over 5,000 physicians and nurses in Army community hospitals and medical centers around the globe. Nurses are able to travel and are able to change geographic location and practice settings without losing seniority.

Since the Army nurse joins the Corps as a commissioned officer, there is no need to go through regular basic training. Instead, the nurse's introduction to the Army is a nine week officer basic orientation course given at the Academy of Health Sciences at Fort Sam Houston, San Antonio, Texas. While at Fort Sam Houston, the nurse attends lectures, conferences, films, and demonstrations that cover everything from military customs to management of mass casualties. Several days are also spent in field nursing practice in a simulated combat environment.

The initial active duty commitment is for three years. At the end of that time, the Army nurse may elect to request to remain on active duty for a short period of time or to apply for a conditional career status. Another option is to return to civilian life and transfer to the Army Reserve. Reserve obligation is five years if the nurse was without prior service when he or she entered the Army Nurse Corps. Reserve duties usually consist of attending meetings one weekend (16 hours) per month, plus two weeks of active duty per year.

A nurse without any previous military experience may join the Army Reserve if he or she has the following qualifications:

1. Be a United States citizen (or have applied for citizenship).

2. Be at least 21 years of age and be able to complete 20 years of service before reaching age 60.

3. Be a graduate of an AD, diploma, or baccalaureate nursing program accredited by an agency recognized by the United States Secretary of Education and acceptable to the Army. (Graduates of AD and diploma programs must have an additional twelve months of nursing experience).

4. Possess a license to practice nursing in any state or the District of Columbia.

5. Be able to meet medical fitness standards.

6. Be able to provide professional references.

Nurses in the Army Reserve have multiple educational opportunities, and continuing education benefits if they successfully complete 20 qualifying years of service.

NAVY.   If you are an RN in good standing and actively engaged in the practice of nursing, you are eligible to apply for a direct appointment into the Navy Nurse Corps. If accepted, you will be appointed an ensign, lieutenant junior grade, or lieutenant, depending upon your education and experience. As a Navy nurse, you will give direct patient care and will also participate in the ongoing informal education of hospital corps personnel.

Navy nurses work in the following clinical areas: general medicine, general surgery, plastic surgery, dental surgery, urology, thoracic surgery, obstetrics and gynecology, psychiatry, neurosurgery, orthopedics, opthalmology, otorhinolaryngology, pediatrics, emergency room, operating room, inservice education, ambulatory care, and critical care units. For the Navy nurse, there is a wide range of continuing education programs available. There is also a two-year nurse-anesthetist course. If accepted into the anesthetist program, the Navy nurse adds, upon its completion, an additional three-year active duty obligation.

For the nurse just starting her naval experience, the three-year tour of active duty begins on the date travel commences to the Naval Officer Education and Training Center in Newport, Rhode Island, for indoctrination. After spending time at a United States facility, the Navy nurse is eligible for overseas assignment.

The qualifications for appointment to the Navy Nurse Corps are:

1. Graduation from an accredited baccalaureate program (this program is preferred, although a limited number of positions are also available for graduates of an accredited nursing school of at least 108 academic weeks' duration, not including vacation periods, with a minimum of twelve months' nursing experience).

2. Be between 20 and 34 years of age to be commissioned.

3. Possess a current license to practice nursing in at least one state, the District of Columbia, or a territory of the United States.

4. Be a citizen of the United States.

5. There are no marriage restrictions. Men and women are eligible.

In the Naval Reserve, qualifications are similar to those for active duty. The main difference is the requirement of a baccalaureate degree and the fact that nurses are accepted in the Reserve up to 40 years of age. There are two Naval Reserve programs; one is a voluntary training unit, in which a nurse receives points toward retirement pay; the other is a paid program. Nurses in the reserve work one night per week or one weekend per month and put in two weeks of active duty every year for up to twenty years. Depending on the nurse's specialty and place of residence, work may be in a naval hospital, civilian hospital, or reserve center. During the two weeks of active duty, assignments are varied and may involve travel and additional training.

AIR FORCE.   In addition to providing traditional nursing care to military personnel and their families, as Army and Navy nurses do, Air Force nurses may also serve as flight nurses or may serve in the aerospace program through their practice in environmental health.

In aeromedical evacuation flights, flight nurses care for thirty to forty litter patients, forty ambulatory patients, or a combination of both. The nursing staff on each aircraft (called C-9 Nightingales) normally consists of five people. Because caring for patients aboard an aircraft is so special, extra training is required before the nurse can wear the wings of a flight nurse. As one Air Force nurse explained, "being a flight nurse is an opportunity I would never have had as a civilian nurse. For me, the hard work and special training were worth it."

Besides this very special area, an Air Force nurse can serve as a nurse anesthetist, a pediatric nurse practitioner, an obstetrics-gynecology nurse practitioner, a nurse-midwife, an operating nurse, or a mental health nurse, as well as the usual clinical specialties. There are also opportunities in hyperboric nursing and research.

The Air Force nurse-midwifery program, established in the early 1970s, was the first in the Department of Defense. Currently there are more than fifty nurse-midwives in the Air Force. Approximately forty are graduates of the nine-month Air Force nurse-midwifery school.

If a nurse fulfills the primary educational requirements, he or she may be commissioned as an Air Force second lieutenant. With additional education or experience, the nurse may enter with a higher rank. Three years of active duty will begin with travel to the professional medical orientation course in Wichita Falls, Texas. The Air Force has a well established internship program to assist first-year nurses with the transition from the beginning practitioner role to that of fully qualified professional.

Basic qualifications for commission in the Air Force Nurse Corps are as follows:

1. Graduate of an accredited school of nursing acceptable to the Surgeon General, United States Air Force.

2. Be at least 18 years of age.

3. Possess current registration in any state or territory of the United States or the District of Columbia.

4. Be a citizen of the United States.

5. Be able to meet physical requirements.

There is also an Air Force Reserves Corps that is open to nurses with or without previous military experience.

Peace Corps

"My first few days were a blur of sand, dirt and flies."

"It was hard to remember that traditional Muslim men never shake a woman's hand."

"We lounged under a tent eating dates and drinking tea. I got my first sense of the vast and empty beauty of the Sahara."

These first impressions of the land of Mauritania were offered by Peace Corps nurses. Two years later, these same volunteers were preparing to leave. They spoke of their difficulty in adapting to and working within a traditional society; the frustrations they felt when the smallest change seemed overwhelming; and how uncomfortable it was when the temperature rose to 120° and the sandstorms continued for days. The dramatic changes that they hoped for in the country's preventive health services program did not happen. However, much of their work did go well; they made many close friends and they learned a great deal about the culture of Mauritania through their first-hand experiences.

Statistically, only one out of every seven applicants becomes a Peace Corps trainee. On the average, three out of four trainees successfully complete training and are selected as volunteers. It is the Peace Corps's goal that only the best-qualified people will serve overseas.

After initial in-country training courses in language, cross-culture, and technical skill building, Peace Corps Volunteer nurses work side-by-side with host-country nurses and health workers within the framework of existing primary health care systems. In this capacity, they may work in professional training institutions as instructors of nurses or they may work in community health centers as trainers of mid-level health personnel, village health workers, and rural extension agents. Training and experience in public health nursing as well as previous experience in informal and formal education is of particular value, although Peace Corps nurses may have a range of educational backgrounds, including graduation from associate degree, diploma, and baccalaureate programs.

Peace Corps volunteers are paid an allowance, usually on a monthly basis, that covers food, clothing, housing, and incidentals. Allowances are based on local living costs and differ from country to country and even within a country.

Host countries request assistance from the Peace Corps, and assignments are made in response to these requests. The Health Department in the government of Western Samoa, for example, requested two volunteers to serve as nurse trainers. One trainer (or teacher) was to work with nursing students in such areas as basic anatomy and physiology or fundamentals of nursing. The other trainer was to teach a six-month post-basic program for midwives. Other duties included supervision and guidance of students in clinical areas of the hospital, evaluation of students' performance, maintaining student records, and participating in programs and on committees concerned with nursing and nursing education. The work, on paper, sounds very much like a nurse's job in the United States. The difference is that medical standards and practices in Western Samoa are not as they are in the United States, and there are language, cultural, and lifestyle differences to which the volunteer must adjust. As in all Peace Corps positions, flexibility, creativity, and patience are necessary traits for the volunteer.

Moving halfway around the globe for an assignment in Liberia, a nurse volunteer is expected to live in a modest mud-brick building with screened windows, wooden shutters, and outdoor latrine and bathing area, and no electricity or running water. Roads are mostly unpaved and are either muddy or dusty, depending on the season. Mail service is at times unreliable. Throughout the two-year experience of providing nursing services to pregnant women and children under five, the Peace Corps nurse will be the only volunteer or expatriate in the town.

The role of a Peace Corps volunteer is not the typical eight-hour-a-day job. It is a two-year commitment that is full-time and person-to-person in a difficult environment. If you can tolerate frustrations, like to work with people as equals, and can cope with living at a basic level in an isolated and often unstructured situation, the Peace Corps can be a rewarding and satisfying assignment. For the right person, it can be the experience of a lifetime.

Public Health Service

From the futuristic world of the National Institutes of Health in Bethesda, Maryland to an Indian reservation in the deserts of New Mexico ... from a cool, green valley in the Tennessee foothills to a crowded inner-city clinic, nurses in the Public Health Service work in a variety of locations serving the Nation's health needs. Virtually every nursing specialty is represented in the Public Health Service and nurses have an opportunity to work with the most advanced, innovative techniques and equipment as well as a chance to experience a cross-cultural health care setting.

The Public Health Service employs through two personnel systems, the civil service and commissioned corps.

If you enter the civil service system, the qualifications you need are determined by the position for which you apply. Grade and salary are based on the education and experience required by the position. Applications can be obtained from your local Federal Jobs Information Centers, listed in your telephone directory.

The Commissioned Corps is an all officer group that serves to meet the needs of the Public Health Service. To qualify as a nurse officer in the corps, you must have at least a BS in nursing from a school or university accredited by the National League for Nursing; be 44 years of age or younger; be a United States citizen; have current licensure; and meet medical standards. For further information on the Commissioned corps system, contact the Department of Health and Human Services (address in appendix).

The top-ranking official in the United States Public Health Service is the surgeon general. In January, 1982, Faye Abdellah, RN, EdD, FAAN, was promoted to deputy surgeon general and became the first nurse and the first woman to hold that post.

Red Cross Nursing

When people think of Red Cross nursing, they often think of disaster services and providing nursing care in some troubled area of the world. Certainly this has been an important aspect of the Red Cross nurse's job since it began over one hundred years ago. But it's by no means the only job a Red Cross nurse is asked to perform.

Nationwide, there are three basic functions of Red Cross nursing: education, disaster relief, and direct services. It's important to realize that for every paid Red Cross staff member an average of 600 persons serve as volunteers. The Red Cross could neither exist nor provide its many services without these volunteers. This is as true in the nursing department as in the other organizational areas.

In educational nursing services, for example, volunteer instructors train volunteer RNs to teach basic courses in home nursing, preparation for parenthood, parenting, and baby-sitting, as well as administering CPR, taking vital signs, and providing health services in times of disaster. For taking the instructor courses, nurses receive continuing education units at the same time that they are serving their communities.

In the area of direct services, Red Cross nurses manage blood pressure clinics and are active in health fairs where free screening services are provided. The Red Cross works under a congressional charter to provide disaster relief. In the department of nursing services, there is a corps of volunteer and paid nurses—most volunteers actively work in critical-care areas in local hospitals or in public health agencies. These nurses are specially trained and ready to help staff emergency aid stations; work in hospitals; shelters, and morgues; or to help set up temporary infirmaries. After the disaster has passed, nurses are used to provide follow-up home visits to victims and their families.

For the past fifteen years, the Red Cross has responded to an annual average of 31,000 disasters to alleviate the suffering of victims. Some of these are local events where response by nurses is minimal. But in the case of widespread catastrophe, there is a skill bank of persons nationwide who may be assigned to a disaster.

Besides the national headquarters in Washington, D.C., there are over 3,000 local units, or chapters, of the American Red Cross. Although most function under the same structure and offer most of the same services, each one is a little different.

Whatever form it takes, wherever humanitarian services are needed, Red Cross workers are there. And nursing services—both on a paid and voluntary basis—are a major aspect of the organization's care and concern.

Project HOPE

"Our work here runs the spectrum of frustration to gratification," says Lisa Forman, HOPE Nurse Educator. "The frustrations, though, seem to melt away when I see the counterpart I trained teaching a less experienced nurse. There is great potential here among the nurses and, for the first time in my life, I'm thrilled at the prospect of losing my job to one of our students."

Susan Griffin, a former HOPE Nurse Educator in Brazil, explains: "This is a very different—very special—kind of nursing. I taught a basic six-week course in nursing fundamentals. There was no testing and no grades were given. In addition to my lectures, the students worked on the wards—with their counterparts—to learn how to give proper nursing care. I also taught classes to large groups of native nurses on various subjects.

"To understand why working in this area was so different, you'd have to know a little of the culture. The people speak Portuguese, and language was occasionally a barrier. The people are very warm and loving. They'd get up right close when talking to you and would love to kiss you on both cheeks in greeting and parting. They would frequently give us gifts, even though you knew they didn't have enough money to feed their families adequately. Formal education was very limited."

Nurses play a vital role in HOPE programs around the world, contributing their knowledge and teaching skills in such countries as

Belize, Brazil, China, Costa Rica, Egypt, Grenada, Guatemala, Jamaica, Panama, Poland, Swaziland, and the United States.

More then 1,200 nurses have served in HOPE's overseas and domestic programs since the Foundation's beginning in 1958. In the year July, 1986 to June, 1987, the organization answered inquiries of 1,534 nurses, 880 of whom will be qualified to work at some time.

Employment service opportunities at Project HOPE, either short (four weeks to three months) or long term (six months or longer), vary with the opening of new programs and with the extension of current programs. Qualifications for positions are program specific and depend on such factors as the defined program request, level of manpower training, culture, language and resources in the country.

Project HOPE is constantly recruiting nurses both for open positions and in anticipation of future needs. The basic requirement is that a nurse possess a BSN and two years clinical experience. Because of the educational nature of most of the programs, however, over 50 percent of the nurses hired have at least a master's degree and significant teaching experience. Although previous international experience is not usually a requirement for positions, it does weigh considerably in a candidate's favor.

Other Opportunities

Nurse missionaries from all faiths may work in mission hospitals or health centers or may serve in an educational or consulting role with native nurses. Whether working in a volunteer or paid capacity, missionary nurses find it particularly satisfying to share their religious beliefs at the same time that they provide nursing services.

What does it take to be a missionary nurse? First, one must be a Christian who is concerned with helping people of other cultures. Some mission boards require a baccalaureate program or a certain amount of prior nursing experience.

For a missionary nurse, the language and surroundings will be foreign, there may be environmental and health hazards, and there will certainly be periods of loneliness. For this reason, physical, mental and spiritual strength are a necessity. Wages are generally low, but the personal rewards, for the right person, are manifold.

The best source for further information is to contact your church's mission board or discuss your plans with the pastor.

Sherut La'am/American Zionist Youth Foundation is an educational nonprofit organization that has no connection with missionary work but does provide an enriching opportunity for young people to travel and live in a different culture.

Sherut La'am serves both the people of Israel and the program participants from abroad who go to work there. Volunteer participants receive room and board in exchange for their work. They also have the opportunity for extensive touring of the country. Participants make their own travel arrangements to Israel.

After three months of Hebrew study (five hours a day, six days a week), placements are made in development towns for a nine-month period. If a person is proficient in Hebrew and has had prior experience in Israel he or she may volunteer for a six-month program. The one-year Sherut La'am program begins in March, July, and October of each year; applications for the six-month program are accepted year round.

Sherut La'am is open to persons 20 to 35 years of age, and all applicants are required to complete an established screening procedure. Independence, creativity, initiative, flexibility, and a sense of humor are helpful characteristics to possess.

CHAPTER 8

Teaching, Research, Administration, Law, Clinical Specialists, Communications

For the student or newly licensed nurse, the idea of such prestigious fields as teaching, research, administration, law or clinical specialist may seem very distant. These are the top positions that pay well and usually offer the greatest degree of autonomy and satisfaction. Relatively few make it to the top, but those who do become decision makers and enjoy a great amount of respect from their peers.

TEACHING

Teaching is the oldest and most influential of nursing's specialities. According to a 1986 survey by the National League for Nursing, there are 17,825 full-time and 5,792 part-time faculty members in RN programs in the United States. Of the full-time faculty members, 13 percent hold doctorates and 75 percent have master's degrees. Of the number of directors or administrators (the top-level position), 57.1 percent had earned a master's degree and 41.8 percent held doctoral degrees. A minimum of a master's degree is recommended for teachers in all nursing programs; doctorates are recommended for deans of collegiate programs and all faculty of graduate programs. With this new standard, there are increasing numbers of teachers returning to school, and the supply of qualified teachers can hardly keep up with the demand.

In the college setting, educators move through the ranks of instructor, assistant or associate professor, professor, and finally dean. The dean of a collegiate nursing program may be called director, administrator, or chairperson.

Patricia Schmidt, RN, EdD, former chairperson of the nursing education department at Palomar Community College in San Marcos, California comments on the role of formal nursing education: "Schools provide structured class time, audiovisual aids, hands-on practice in the laboratory and clinical setting, and bibliographies for independent reading and research. The ultimate responsibility for learning, however, lies with the student. The school acts as a facilitator, but in the final analysis a student will get out of the program what he or she puts into it. Education is an independent search—tests will determine if that search has been fruitful."

These may sound like harsh words from this warm and enthusiastic nurse who "loves teaching" and has led many students into fulfilling careers, but Dr. Schmidt is aware of the realities of her profession. One of the realities is that nurses must take greater responsibility for their learning.

Doris Schoneman is assistant professor of nursing at Marquette University in Milwaukee, Wisconsin. One of five faculty members in the department of community health nursing, Ms. Schoneman is responsible for educating students in both lecture and field experiences. She teaches a freshman introductory nursing class and a junior level course on family. The greatest amount of time, however, is spent working with seniors who are gaining field experience in community health.

"I spend 45 to 50 hours a week in my position but my day to day responsibilities often vary. Usually, I start in the morning with the eight senior students who are gaining practical experience in community health. We spend about an hour discussing some topic before the students go out in the field. Field experiences can be home visits, blood pressure screening clinics, screening clinics for senior citizens, or assessment visits at a day care center.

"I accompany the students on some of their home visits. For many students, this is their first experience outside the hospital. They are initially nervous about home visiting, but become more comfortable with each visit. I act as a role model on these initial visits and often conduct part of the interview to show the student how to do it. I feel that being a positive role model is the most important aspect of my work. If I'm not enthusiastic about nursing, I can't expect my students to be that way. It's a pleasure and privilege to be so much a part of a student's life and to see that student grow as the weeks go by.

"Many students begin their community health experience with the notion that it will be interesting but will probably not be of great benefit to their careers since many plan to take positions in acute care after graduating. But students continually tell me, at the end of the rotation, that they became much more family focused after completing community health. I had a student, for example, who was scheduled to make a home visit with a patient who had just been admitted to the hospital. She said, 'I guess I'll cancel the visit this week since my client's in the hospital.'

"I asked her, 'Is there anything else you might do for your client?'

"She thought for a moment then answered, 'I guess I could visit her in the hospital. And, you know, her husband has a lot of feelings about this. Maybe I should make a home visit after all.'

"I was really proud of this student's decision because she was realizing that in all of nursing, you have to care about the entire family and not just the individual client. The student made the home visit and it was beneficial to both the client's husband and to the student."

In addition to working directly with the students, Ms. Schoneman works on various committees in the college of nursing and the university. She also serves as an advisor to the student nurse organization and is active in the American Nurses' Association. Then there's research, preparation of class material and grading papers.

This is Schoneman's second year of teaching and it's a big change from her previous assignments in community health and ambulatory care. "I like the flexibility in my present position. If, for example, I need to go to the library to research a subject, I can freely do that. It's an expectation in academia that we keep up on things. If I were practicing at a hospital or an agency there might not be time to delve into subjects in which I have an interest."

Ms. Schoneman obtained her BSN degree from University of Iowa and her MS from University of Wisconsin at Milwaukee. Before taking her present position, she worked as a staff public health nurse, nursing director of a county health department and director of three out-patient clinics. "The pressures—for me—are much less in teaching than they were in administration. Of course the salary is not as good but the flexibility and freedom that I enjoy is well worth the trade-off."

Some drawbacks? "The community health rotation is only eight weeks and I often would like to work with the students longer. I know that many of them are capable of learning and doing more, and that can be frustrating. Also there's a constant challenge in education to make sure that the students we graduate are adequately prepared to contribute in a health care system that's continually changing. On a personal level, there's a need for me to complete my PhD and, while I'm teaching, find the time to keep up my clinical skills. Some faculty members have joint appointments so that they can continue keeping up their skills at the same time that they're teaching."

Ms. Schoneman feels that the most important quality for someone interested in teaching is that he or she enjoy nursing and be able to project that love and passion to students. "A teacher should also enjoy working with students and helping them develop their full potential. It's essential of course that a teacher be competent and have a good practice base. In addition, universities require a minimum master's degree and, for the top positions especially, a PhD is required."

Ms. Schoneman concludes, "I was fortunate to work as a teaching assistant and research assistant when I was completing my masters. That helped me to see the possibilities for teaching. In addition, I worked with several professors who served as my mentors. They were able to provide needed advice and assistance. As to the future, I plan to continue teaching and perhaps combine that role with research. It's very satisfying to work with students and help them become the best nurses they can be."

RESEARCH

Marcella Z. Davis, RN, DNSc, FAAN, is one of the pioneers in the field of nursing research. At a time when few nurses were involved in research, she received a Fulbright Research Scholarship in 1955 to conduct a study in Great Britain. Her research career has continued since that auspicious beginning. She is a Fellow of the American Academy of Nursing (FAAN), has served on the faculty of several prominent university schools of nursing, has published numerous articles and two books, and has spoken to many prestigious groups and organizations in the United States and abroad. She just completed a 12 year position as associate chief of nursing service for research at the Veterans Administration Medical Center in San Diego and associate professor-in-residence in the department of community medicine at the University of California, San Diego and is now teaching doctoral students in Ethnographic Research at the University of San Diego.

While at the Veterans Administration Medical Center, Dr. Davis spent 90 percent of her time actively involved in nursing research. She would meet with nurse clinicians, review materials, set up the design of a project, collect and analyze the data, report her findings in the literature, and help initiate change based on her research within the work setting.

Davis also brought converts into the research fold. She was readily accessible to the staff nurses, but did require that nurses make an appointment so that her own work day was not disrupted. As Davis explains, "The nurses were encouraged to come and discuss their project ideas with me. Many times these were vague notions that were swirling around in their heads. I could help them formulate and organize their ideas and together we could create a well-designed project. My position in the institution conferred legitimacy to clinical nurses engaged in their practice-based research. It would have been difficult, if not impossible, for many clinical nurses to engage in research activity without this legitimization. That should not be surprising, since nurses are hired to provide patient care services— research activity is not yet fully accepted, by most institutions and by many nurses, as a legitimate part of a nurse's role."

Because of Dr. Davis, there are now a number of nurses at the San Diego Veterans Administration Medical Center who "think research." The typical research that clinical nurses are engaged in is based on their day-to-day practice and focuses on ways of improving care to patients as well as on problems that may affect the patient's family under the stress of serious illness. For example, as a result of one study of the relatives of newly diagnosed cancer patients, nurse-led support groups for these family members are now a routine part of the hospital services. Because of another nurse's study, delivery of care in one area of the hospital has been changed. Emergency room patients, before they leave the hospital, now see a registered nurse and not a clerk, as was the former practice, to be certain their questions are answered and to review their treatment plan.

When Dr. Davis first took on the job at the medical center in 1975, most nurses in the clinical setting were unfamiliar with research and some were skeptical about its application to their work situation. To familiarize the staff with this relatively new concept, Davis initiated monthly nursing research work sessions. At these meetings, some nurses expressed an interest in knowing more about the relevance of research to nursing practice. Some nurses were also interested in learning about a nurse's responsibilities in regard to obtaining informed consent from patients who were research subjects. A few nurses were looking for encouragement and assistance in working on their own research projects. It was this last group with whom Davis spent the most time. These nurses were allowed time away from the clinical work area to perform research activities and were given other incentives to carry out their work. It was not always smooth sailing, though, because some nurses looked on research activity as "playing" or saw the work as an extension of the so-called physician/male role rather than the nurse/female role.

Not all research nurses have the freedom and independence that Dr. Davis enjoyed at the Veterans Medical Center in San Diego. She explains: "The Veterans Administration, back in the early sixties, pioneered in nursing research by establishing clinically based research positions for doctorally prepared nurses. The more typical location for doctorally prepared nurses, who may or may not have conducted research, was in university schools of nursing. There is a trend now for clinical institutions to hire research nurses. It makes sense, since this is the area where nurses need to investigate problems in patient care and to effect change. However, in some hospital settings, the research position has become heavily diluted with educational and administrative responsibilities, thereby impairing the efforts of the nurse researcher to seriously conduct research of any consequence."

In October 1987, Dr. Davis presented a paper at the ANA sponsored *International Nursing Research Conference* in Washington, D.C. The paper was an extension of an eighteen month study of 28 persons (15 men and 13 women), half of whom were veterans who received health services and care from the Veterans Medical Center. Most were aged 85 and older—a population about whom very little is known yet that is the fastest increasing age group among the elderly and the population in general. The work involved interviews to determine how the aged person perceives himself or herself. Davis found that chronological age is but one among many factors that defines who and what the older person is. The implications for her colleagues? "Health professionals in both hospital and community settings are in a highly advantageous position to further the efforts of the long-lived individual to be viewed as more than his advanced age by creating an opportunity in social interaction with them, that offer a chance for the expression of other facets of their identity. This recommendation is simple, it's obvious, and it's feasible. It requires as a start, that we ask about the long-lived individual, 'who is this person other than the old woman/man I see before me?'"

What does it take to be a research nurse? Besides being a creative thinker and having the tools to follow the research process, a nurse in this specialty needs to possess an abundance of patience and persistence. She also needs to be proficient in speaking and writing. All of these skills are not obtained when the nurse receives her doctoral degree, but that credential is usually a requirement for a full-time research nurse.

In tracing Marcella Davis's background, one is impressed with the magnitude of her accomplishments. A graduate of a New Jersey diploma program, she worked for a short time as a psychiatric nurse at Bellevue Hospital before contracting tuberculosis. After spending three years at a sanatorium in upstate New York, she received a New York tuberculosis and health scholarship and obtained a BS degree at New York University. Following two years of clinical experience, Davis continued her education at Columbia University, where she received an MS degree in psychiatric nursing. Next she held a position as assistant professor at the University of Maryland School of Nursing. In 1955, she received a Fulbright Award, which permitted her to teach and conduct research in Great Britain. When she returned to the University of Maryland, Davis's life took a different turn. She married, had a child, and taught part-time at Columbia University for two years. She and her husband (a professor of sociology) took faculty positions at the University of California at San Francisco and stayed in the area for fifteen years. It was at this institution that Davis obtained her doctorate in nursing science.

When Dr. Davis was at the Veterans Hospital, a typical research day involved reading, interviewing, or writing as she pursued the various phases of a research project. "I could spend the full eight hours a day, five days a week, on research. If there were other demands on my time—for example, a conference with a nurse or the once-a-month committee meetings that I attended—I tried to do my research work in the morning hours when I work best. The days went by very quickly and the work was always stimulating."

More and more nurses are joining the ranks of Dr. Davis and other researchers. Their pioneering efforts in this area are already doing much to improve nursing care and to enhance the status of the profession.

ADMINISTRATION AND MANAGEMENT

"The position of director of nursing in a modern hospital has been compared to the position of a football coach. In his job as the coach (director), he is responsible to the owners (administration), and the fans (patients), and the players (nurses and doctors). When anything gets out of sync, the first one asked to leave is the football coach (director)."

This analogy comes from a nursing administrator who had a great influence on the career of Director Joyce Foy of San Diego's Pomerado Hospital. Foy, who was appointed to her present post six years ago, has had a long career in administration and is aware of the stresses that are inherent in this type of position. Among her peers, burnout and high job turnover are not uncommon.

All nursing administrators have to answer to many bosses. Nursing guidelines are set down by the Joint Commission on Accreditation of Healthcare Organizations (JCAHO), and individual state laws require certain criteria. California law, for example, requires that there be one nurse for every two patients in an intensive care unit. In addition to these restraints, there are decisions made by the hospital's board of directors and by the attending physicians, and there are demands and input from consumer groups and nursing organizations. The list is endless. To work in the administrative milieu, a nursing director must understand management methods, political systems, and relationships within the health care system and the community. In all these areas, she must think not only of present needs but also of future hospital needs. It is a top-level position that pays top dollar.

Director Foy comments, "Different nurses make good directors in different hospitals. In any situation, though, I think it's important that administrators be tactful in dealing with others. Personality does enter into this type of job. My opinion is that a person who has the ability to relax and relate well with people will do better than an authoritarian type of individual. In addition, a director should be organized and yet flexible."

The 130-bed Pomerado Hospital where Foy works is one of two district hospitals. An executive director oversees the two separate administrations. Foy's position as nursing director is on the level of an assistant administrator; she reports directly to the hospital administrator. As is true in all hospitals, the nursing service at Pomerado is the largest department in the hospital and commands the biggest budget. Foy's position therefore carries a considerable amount of authority and a great deal of responsibility. "The director of nursing has no peer within the hospital, so the contacts we have with other nursing administrators are very important. The Nursing Administrators Council, part of the Hospital Council, is made up of all nursing directors in this area. We meet regularly and discuss various problem-solving ideas. It's a very important networking group."

Nurse Foy is required to attend many meetings, such as those with medical staff committee members, other department heads, and management personnel. In the nursing area, she meets weekly with the head nurses on each unit and twice a month with the supervisors, head nurses, and other management-level nurses. Four times a year, or more frequently, Director Foy holds a nursing forum meeting where all nurses, full-time and per diem, meet with her and take part in a free exchange of ideas and discussion of mutual problems.

Foy has recently hired a hospital pool of per diem nurses who can be called in the event of nurse absence or increased patient census. This will diminish the hospital's previous dependence on agency nurses.

One project in which Foy is deeply involved is setting up the district's OPPUS (ON-LINE Palomar Pomerado User-Designed System) computer system. This is an integrated system with a single data base that will connect all operations in the hospital district, including two hospitals, a home health agency, multiple outreach programs, a blood bank, two skilled nursing facilities, hospice, and the corporate offices.

There will be computer terminals at each patient's bedside. These terminals will provide instant access to timely patient data collection, patient demographics, activities, medical histories, orders written and executed by all care providers. The terminals will be utilized by the nurses to do patient charting. The nurse will perform her assessment of the patient, enter this information into the computer and a nursing diagnosis will be made. A nursing care plan will then be provided from which the nurse can select the appropriate intervention to fit the individual patient's needs.

Besides her hospital duties, Nurse Foy also serves on an advisory board for a local AD nursing program and from time to time is invited to speak to or become involved with various community groups.

Director Foy is a graduate of a Canadian diploma program. She obtained her BSN and MS in nursing administration at California State University, Los Angeles. She was vice-president for nursing at a 360-bed hospital in Los Angeles and was also patient care administrator for a large health maintenance organization. Foy also worked in other hospitals and in industry and taught in an AD nursing program before joining the staff at Pomerado Hospital.

"There is an abundance of paperwork in this position, and that's not a chore I particularly like. I may be tied up with meetings all day and afterwards I might want to get out and be on the units. But there's always papers that must be read or signed. However, I try to interact with the nurses as much as possible, since I get a great amount of personal satisfaction in being involved with them and their concerns. One of the best parts of an administrative job is being the catalyst for producing growth in others. At the hospital where I previously worked, it was a privilege to teach and work with a bright staff nurse who moved through the ranks and is now director.

"It's very gratifying to come into an organization and help make things run smoothly while still maintaining the individual identity of staff members. It's also a great challenge!"

NURSE ATTORNEY

"The nursing process and the legal process are very similar," says New York Nurse Attorney Cynthia Northrop. "In both nursing and law, you have to be able to quickly identify and assess a problem, then apply the necessary principles."

"There's another parallel in these helping professions," continues Ms. Northrop. "Nurses historically learned their skills in the hospital setting while lawyers spent their apprenticeship in law firms. For lawyers, entry into practice has been resolved—that is, a law degree is generally required. But for nurses, this is an issue that still needs to be worked out."

Cynthia Northrop has been a nurse attorney for seven years. She is a member of the Maryland and New York bars and currently practices law in New York City. Her time is split between the law practice, teaching, giving workshops, and writing.

Northrop's legal clients are nurses or occasionally home health agencies, health departments or nursing organizations. "One day this week I received four calls from nurses. One was a nurse who was accused of abusing a patient and was going to be reprimanded by the Board of Nursing. Another was from a nurse who was attacked by a nurse's aide. Still another nurse—this one a supervisor—had been ordered to work weekends and wondered if she could challenge this. And finally, a nurse with a drug problem was being threatened with loss of his license. I'll probably represent these four nurses and set up individual appointments to discuss their problems in greater detail.

What I'll do is put the facts together, find out what the nurses want to do and what we'll be able to do. Many times, all that's needed is a neutral third party to give legal information and negotiate the problem. These cases won't necessarily go to court. Maybe a letter or phone call will be sufficient. Sometimes, however, a case can go on for two to five years and can become more complicated. I often collaborate with other nurse attorneys.

"Unfortunately, I often need to represent nurses who are impaired with drugs or alcohol. As part of my efforts to help these clients, a number of nurses and I recently organized a nurse recovery group in New York City. It was long overdue!"

In addition to her law practice, Ms. Northrop is an adjunct associate professor at Teachers College, Columbia University. One day a week, she teaches a graduate-level course in legal issues in nursing through the Department of Nursing Education.

Besides these activities, the nurse attorney teaches workshops across the country at universities, health facilities and for continuing education companies. On an average, Northrop teaches two or three workshops a week. She also writes a column for two nursing journals—*Nursing Life* and *Nursing Outlook.* In April 1987, Northrop's book, *Legal Issues in Nursing* (coauthored with nurse attorney Mary Kelly) was published by C.V. Mosby Co.

Cynthia Northrop's days are obviously full and the most difficult part of her job is keeping up with such a hectic schedule. "A nurse may call today, for example, and say that her hearing is scheduled for tomorrow. I have to decide quickly if I can juggle things around to help this person or if there's a chance I can get the time of the hearing changed. Sometimes I think that a hearing will last for an hour but instead it takes six hours.

"Mostly, though, I like the challenges of my work and I especially like being able to provide a support system for other nurses. For most nurse attorneys, nursing was their first love and they like to help and support their peers. It's especially gratifying to be able to help nurses who are having disputes over control of their practices."

What career path did Nurse Northrop follow to get where she is today? After receiving her bachelor's degree in nursing from Columbia Union College in Maryland, she worked on a pre- and postsurgical floor in a general hospital and then worked as a public health nurse for a health department. After receiving her MS in community health nursing at the University of Maryland, Ms. Northrop worked as a clinical nurse specialist in community health. "It was my work with child abuse cases that led to my interest in law. I often had to testify in court about clients and I was interested in the legal aspects of this and other public health matters."

Ms. Northrop taught courses in community health at the University of Maryland School of Nursing at the same time that she was attending law school at the University of Baltimore. She was on the faculty at the University of Maryland for nine years before moving to New York City.

The future? Ms. Northrop hopes to continue to build her law practice and cut back on the workshops. The nurse attorney is quick to point out that there are many opportunities in her field. "Although there's a glut of lawyers, there are not enough lawyers with a background in health care. And more and more, women are becoming lawyers and better positions are opening up for them. For someone interested in this field, I would suggest that they get a strong educational background. A BSN is probably best because you need a bachelor's degree as entry into law school. It's very important to practice nursing for a time before going to law school.

"In order to be successful, a nurse attorney needs to be assertive, organized, and knowledgeable. She should enjoy problem solving and have excellent writing skills."

Cynthia Northrop was the Founder and Past President of the American Association of Nurse Attorneys, Inc. This organization has a membership of over 300 men and women. Members' practices include personal injury, risk management, general hospital and insurance law, health care regulation, nursing practice, teaching in nursing or law schools, hospital administration and general civil and administrative law. Nurse attorneys earn an average salary of $40,000–50,000 per year. One recent survey of 60 nurse attorneys found a range of $24,000 per year for a new attorney to $140,000 per year for an established attorney in private practice.

Combining nursing and the law is certainly not for everyone. But as the need for legal-health services continues to increase, the law will become an even more attractive option for the bright and ambitious nurse who wants to practice her profession in a very special way.

CLINICAL SPECIALIST

Since the early 1960s, the clinical nurse specialist (CNS) has assumed an increasingly significant role in providing quality patient care. Working directly with patients or working in a consultant role with other nurses, this nurse is a specialist in one particular area of nursing (for example, medicine, surgery, or pediatrics). The CNS may also work in a more narrowly defined specialty, such as rehabilitation or oncology. There are approximately 24,000 CNSs in the nation.

The CNS is the expert in making a nursing diagnosis and prescribing the appropriate nursing action. She makes both short-term and long-term goals for patient care. The advanced knowledge that a clinical specialist possesses is usually obtained through study on the master's level.

"Most clinical specialists divide their time between the areas of practice (working directly with patients), education (of nursing staff and other health workers), and research and administration," says Bonnie Allbaugh, a clinical specialist for medical nursing at Meriter Hospital in Madison, Wisconsin. "But every CNS builds her own practice, depending on the particular institution's areas of greatest need and the nurse's own interests and expertise. I started out seven years ago, for example, as a specialist in cardiac nursing but now most of my practice is devoted to working with diabetic patients and this has become my area of specialty."

What is a "typical day" like for Allbaugh? "I have no 'typical day' but my pattern is usually to go on nursing unit rounds first. I'm connected with five medical units. I carry a regular case load of patients and I'm also on call to the other units such as surgical or specialty areas. I carry a beeper and respond to problems as they arise. I also work in the outpatient diabetic clinic two days per week.

"Although my usual work time is 8:00 to 5:30, Monday through Friday, that can get blown to the wind. For one thing, I share call (with another CNS) for patients in the home IV therapy program. If problems arise on evenings or week-ends—and that's usually when problems do occur—I am available by phone to help work things out.

"There's lots of patient teaching in this position. I'm working now with a diabetic woman who is blind and wants to be independent and give her own insulin. She of course needs special equipment and has special needs. It's a great challenge!

"Another patient is a seven-year-old boy who suffers from osteo-myelitis (a bone disease) and needs six weeks of antibiotic IV therapy at home. Within a week of being home, the boy was giving his own IV antibiotic medicine, flushing the catheter and changing his dress-ing—with parent supervision. He's amazing!

"In still other cases, I may work with the primary nurse so that she can be a more effective teacher. It just depends on what works best for everyone concerned.

"I also teach classes to groups of employees and, in the administrative line, chair committees and sit in on meetings. Most of my research time involves quality assurance or doing studies to determine if nursing care is adequate and appropriate. In addition to these activities, another specialist and I have a small private consulting business with other hospitals."

Allbaugh is active in a number of nursing organizations. A member of the Wisconsin Nurses' Association, she was a board member from 1983 to 1985, vice-president from 1985 to 1987, and will serve as president until 1989. She's also a member of the Nursing Diagnosis Association of North America and does legislative work on the state level for the American Diabetes Association. In 1982, Allbaugh received a grant from Sigma Theta Tau (nursing honorary) to conduct research on "Evaluating the Effectiveness of Preoperative Teaching for Open Heart Surgery."

What path did Allbaugh follow to get to the responsible position she now holds? A graduate of a midwestern diploma program, she received her baccalaureate and master's degrees from University of Wisconsin at Madison. She is certified as a diabetic educator by the American Association of Diabetic Educators (AADE) and will soon be taking the ANA medical-surgical certification exam.

Before becoming a clinical specialist, Allbaugh worked as a staff nurse in medical-surgical, critical care, and public health nursing. She was director of nursing in a small hospital for one and a half years. "It's absolutely essential that a CNS have a broad background in clinical practice. You first need to become an expert generalist before becoming a specialist.

"I learned many of the skills that I use now from other clinical specialists. We have a strong peer group and that's important. But learning is also an individual responsibility—in order to be credible, a clinical specialist must constantly keep up with current practice."

The best part of being a CNS? "The flexibility and variety. One day I may be working with patients, on another day I may be teaching a class or be involved with administrative tasks. It's also exciting to be able to work with a number of different patients and be able to move from one unit to another.

"But the flip side of all this flexibility is having to juggle the various responsibilities and set priorities. A person who likes and needs a lot of structure wouldn't work well as a clinical specialist. Some days I may have nothing scheduled on my calendar but I'm not able to accomplish everything I'd like to. The lack of routine and constant interruptions are part of this specialty. You also need to be extremely skilled as a nurse and not be afraid to interact with physicians and other health personnel. Being assertive is an important personality trait."

The position of clinical nurse specialist is the top rung on the clinical ladder and the position carries a lot of responsibility as well as a lot of power to make changes. For the right person, like Bonnie Allbaugh, it can be very satisfying.

COMMUNICATIONS

Barbara Huttmann is the author of *Code Blue* and *The Patient's Advocate*; Alice Kahn wrote *My Life as a Gal*. Both of these authors are RNs and they speak from a point of view that's refreshingly different from that of their writing peers.

Kathleen Huggins, RN, MS, is a perinatal nurse who wrote *The Nursing Mother's Companion* (Harvard Common Press). Huggins explains how her popular book came about: "I was working with a breast-feeding client in one of the clinics and was helping her over some trouble spots. After we talked she said, 'You have so many ideas that aren't in any of the books that are now on the market. You should write a book yourself.'

"I went home with that thought still in my head. When I told my husband, he thought it was a great idea. The next day I wrote an outline; then, in the following weeks, I wrote the first two chapters and had a nurse editor look it over. It took four months to find a publisher and nine months to write the book. I wrote every day—in long hand—and had someone else put it on the word processor. It was a lonely time while I was writing but, at the same time, it was a satisfying project."

Huggins's book could be called "user friendly" because the reader can look up a breast-feeding problem and find a quick solution. "I wrote it in the style of a 'Fix Your Car Manual' and also have 'survival guides.'" Because Huggins had so much experience at trouble shooting for nursing mothers, she was a "natural" to write *The Nursing Mother's Companion*. Her next book will be a manual for nurses on home phototherapy (therapy carried out at home for jaundiced newborns).

Many nurses are required to write professional articles or consumer instructions as part of their work responsibilities. But a few nurses have moved beyond this on-the-job writing to take their place alongside other journalists and popular writers. Combining a love for writing and an expertise in nursing and health care can be a winning combination and a very satisfying career choice.

Two of the most important qualities for a writer are discipline and organization. Interestingly enough, these are the very qualities that often spell success for a nurse. Again, by virtue of their work, nurses are frequently in touch with "experts" and have ready access to medical libraries. Research is the cornerstone of credibility.

Nurses are also in the mainstream of humanity. They are privileged to be present at birth and death; at times of joy and sorrow. These experiences and the emotions that they produce are what make stories live—and sell.

There's a big market for health articles and not enough people to write them well. More and more, nurses have taken on the job of communicator—with patients, families, other health workers. To be a writer, it's just a question of putting down the information in a useable form and marketing the finished product.

For years, nurses have suffered from bad press. There have been a number of recent studies that point out the unrealistic and negative picture that the public has of nursing and nurses. If there are enough excellent articles by writers with RN after their name, it can have a powerful effect in changing the nurse's image.

E'Louise Ondash enjoyed a fifteen-year career as an RN before becoming a full-time journalist with the Escondido (California) *Times-Advocate*. A diploma graduate, Ondash was attending school and working part-time when she decided to try her hand at freelance writing. "I met the editor of *Senior Life* and thought I would like to write for the local magazine since I could combine my writing skills with a knowledge of gerontology. I wrote down some ideas and the editor liked them. That began my freelance career, although I continued to work in a physician's office part-time while I was writing for the magazine. Four years ago, the *Times-Advocate* was looking for feature writers and for six months I worked part-time before being hired as a full-time staff writer." Ondash writes features on all subjects but particularly likes writing on health matters. She recently wrote a large feature on the local nursing shortage that was well received.

Ondash feels that her nursing experience was excellent preparation for conducting interviews. "I'm not as threatened as some other writers are when I have to go to a person's home for an interview or gather facts from a health expert. As a nurse, I had to interview people under much more stressful situations."

Ms. Ondash would eventually like to be a health writer for a large newspaper and feels that her background could be the ticket for that position. "Because I don't have a journalism degree, I would have to sell a large newspaper on the notion that I have something that no one else has. That unique 'something' would be my background in nursing and my knowledge of health and medicine."

To be a successful nurse writer, you must learn the necessary skills. Join a writing group or attend a writing class through a local university. Learn how to write a good query letter and how to package your manuscript so it looks professional. Propose an article to a nursing journal and then, once published, consider moving into the mainstream publications. You can find out where to send articles and book proposals by reading *Writer's Market* (Writer's Digest Books).

Writing is a skill that improves with practice so write regularly and have faith that you will succeed. According to nurse writer Kathleen Huggins, "The rewards of your finished product far exceed the time and effort."

CHAPTER 9

New Trends in Nursing

THE ROLE OF THE MALE NURSE

Throughout this book, I have usually used the pronoun "she" when referring to a nurse. That's because 97 percent of nurses are women.

Historically, though, men preceded women into nursing. In times of war and plague, men have cared for the sick and the wounded. Even after public hospitals came into being, men gave much of the nursing care until the time of Florence Nightingale. Then, as Nightingale-type nursing schools spread, nursing became a women's profession. According to the National Male Nurse Association, in 1910 men made up 7.4 percent of the nursing force, in 1920, 3.7 percent, and from 1930 to 1960, 1.6 percent. In 1963, the figure had risen to 2.1 percent, and it's now estimated that 3 percent or approximately 50,000 nurses are men. According to a 1985 survey by the National League for Nursing, 5.7 percent of newly licensed nurses were men (5.6 percent of graduates of baccalaureate programs, 6.1 percent of graduates of associate degree programs, and 4.5 percent of graduates of diploma programs). The upward trend for men in nursing is obvious and can be traced to several factors.

The stereotype of "male jobs" and "female jobs" is gradually losing hold. As more men become nurses, secretaries, teachers, and telephone operators, more women are becoming physicians, engineers, and police officers. In these days of liberation, there's more of an emphasis on the best person for the job, rather than the best man or best woman.

Schools of nursing have changed. The traditional three-year diploma program was set up for women, and, with few exceptions, men were not allowed. Just as many minority, handicapped, and older students were shut out, there was not a place for the male student nurse either. Today, the AD programs provide inexpensive, convenient nursing education for all members of the community. And baccalaureate programs find it relatively easy to admit men to the fold.

Nursing, which means "to nourish, to support, and to give of oneself," has always been associated with women generally and mothers specifically. It has traditionally been accepted that a nurse provides the mother image. But modern nursing challenges this theory. Nursing today is not just white uniforms and warm smiles. The work is technical, highly skilled, physically demanding, and suitable to both sexes. Men are still sometimes more willing to make a career

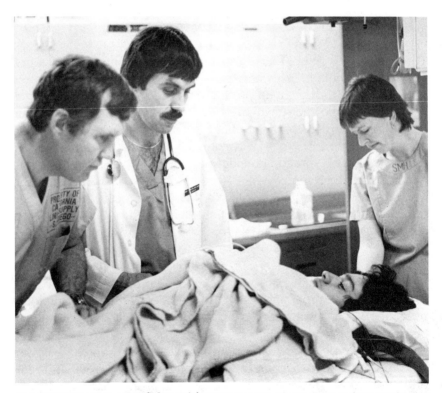

An emergency team in action (left to right) trauma surgeon, trauma nurse, and X-ray technician. *(Photo by Peter James McCracken, Courtesy Scripps Memorial Hospital)*

commitment than women. At this critical time, nursing needs serious practitioners—men and women.

Nursing, as a career, offers many advantages that appeal to members of both sexes. Flexibility, opportunity for advancement, satisfaction in being able to perform a needed service are just some of the advantages. All these have been mentioned before and they can apply to men as well as women.

Robert Salibene is administrator of a 192-bed skilled nursing facility in St. Petersburg, Florida. He has combined his skills in nursing and management to attain the position he holds. His goals and ambitions are now firm in his mind, although it wasn't always that way.

Salibene was a Marine in Vietnam and was active in the peace movement of the 1960s. He obtained a BS in psychology at the State University of New York at Albany. After college, Salibene worked as a respiratory therapist at the Albany Medical Center. Thinking he would like to become a nurse anesthetist, he attended the AD nursing program at Maria College. Once out of school, he found that it was a closed market for nurse anesthetists in that area, so he did psychiatric nursing and moved into a position of supervision. Salibene then obtained an MS in health services management in California. He worked in utilization review for two years and took his nursing home board exams in order to become a nursing home administrator. His goal is to continue in administrative positions, and he hopes to effect some changes for nursing. Salibene, married to another RN, is very honest about the profession he has chosen: "It may be that males are more aggressive, but I think it's really that female nurses have been too passive for too many years. Now, with the women's movement, with women becoming primary breadwinners and with inflation, more women need to improve their salaries. Nurses are often put in a position of feeling guilty when asking for compensation. That isn't right. Also a baccalaureate nurse spends at least $20,000 for his or her education, then has to take continuing education. If she's not going to be compensated and is going to be treated like a handmaiden by the physician, then why do it? Changes need to be made.

"For men interested in nursing, I would suggest they get some exposure with a limited commitment. Either work as a volunteer or an orderly in a hospital or nursing home and see if this is what you like. Then go the AD route and use this as a stepping stone to advance your career. A friend of mine got an AD in nursing and now works in a medical supply house. He makes more money there than he'd ever make in a traditional nursing job."

It has been said that male nurses need to feel very secure in their masculinity, because they'll be continually questioned about it. The Male Nurse Association states, "The stereotype traditionally associated with the males who become nurses usually embodies one of two negative concepts: either he is 'queer' or he is 'power driven' and wants a top position in a field where he can dominate. No doubt there are male nurses who fit these stereotypes, just as there are women nurses who fit them."

Many of the thousands of Vietnam veterans who were medical corpsmen in the armed forces entered nursing. While serving their country, they found they liked medical work but, for various reasons, were not interested in medical school. One of these veterans now serves as a nurse with an emergency medical helicopter team. He had this to say about being a male nurse: "Many times when we're transporting a patient from the field to the hospital, the emergency room physician will approach me first for a report—that's especially true if the physician is a woman. I have yet to meet any prejudice because I'm a man."

Men have been well received in areas of psychiatry, community health, male genitourinary units, orthopedic units, intensive care units, and occupational health. In all fairness, however, there's no reason why men can't be an asset in every nursing specialty.

Ask a female nurse how many male RNs there are on staff and she can usually give you a figure right away. At Pioneer's Memorial Hospital in Brawley, California, there are ten male nurses on staff.

One of these nurses, Juan Mendez, belongs to two minority groups. He is a male nurse and also a Mexican-American. Mendez is presently director of staff development and prior to that was supervisor of the hospital's mental health unit.

If anyone has a success story to tell, it's Juan Mendez. Coming from a family of eleven children, he didn't have the benefits of a positive male role model. But his mother, in her late forties and with a sixth-grade education, went into an LVN program and finished. She supported the family on her nursing salary. Mendez explains, "I flunked out of high school and had very low self-esteem. Everybody gave up on me except my mother. I went into the service and finally got myself together. I took courses and got good grades. After completing the LVN program ten years ago, I began at Pioneer's Memorial in the mental health unit. I joined the LVN-to-RN program, and a year after my license, became supervisor of the unit. For me and my family, this has been the impossible dream. I'm very proud to be an RN and plan to continue my education. I enjoy what I do at the hospital and want to be the best that I can be."

For many men working in the nursing field, this is just the right career choice. And if it is true that one of the problems of nursing is that it's a woman's profession in a society that's dominated by men, then all nurses should welcome the men into their ranks. Most women do.

Michael Johnson is a nurse entrepreneur who started his Seattle-based company—Consulting Opinion, Inc.—in 1984. As an expert on home health care and aging, he now works with new and existing health care agencies in policy and procedure development so that they can become compliant with federal, state or local standards. "One of my clients is an HMO that has contracted with me to assist in the development of a long-term care policy for their Medicare enrollees," says Johnson. "This is a long-term project and I spend one to two days a week with the organization. I even have my own office there."

Johnson has contracts with other agencies and sometimes finds that juggling various assignments can be a problem. "This is one of the biggest pressures in having your own business. I can work from 30 to 60 hours per week. But some months it seems that everyone wants results at the same time. However, the greater flexibility and the variety more than compensate for an occasional hectic schedule. Nurse entrepreneurs have to be highly organized and very disciplined. When you leave a structured position, you also leave a structured work schedule behind. You have to rebuild that schedule and keep on top of things if you want to be a success."

Johnson has always had an interest in long-term health care. He earned a BSN from University of Washington, then worked in home health care for several years before returning to school to complete a master's degree in Social Work. From 1980 to 1984, Johnson was the director of a hospital-based home health agency and later the director of professional services at a large visiting nurse association. When he first started his consulting business, Johnson worked part-time for a year as a field nursing instructor in community health at University of Washington. "In the beginning, when you're building your practice, a nurse entrepreneur often needs a part-time position. I also found it helpful to talk with other consultants to see how much they charged for their services. As my expertise and efficiency increases, I feel that I'm worth more and can charge accordingly.

"I start all assignments with a contract and try to be specific about what the agency wants and what I can provide. Most assignments take six months to a year to complete. I usually charge an hourly fee with a stop limit—what that means is that the total bill won't go over a certain amount without renegotiating with management. Of course, everyone thinks that when you have your own business, you make a lot of money. That's not necessarily true. There are no group benefits and you have to pay more in taxes. And of course you always have to be negotiating to get more assignments. But, for me, the trade-off is worth it when I consider I'm making my own future."

Johnson belongs to a number of professional organizations and finds that, over the years, the support and expertise of peers has been very helpful. He is a member of Senior Services of Washington (a state organization) and two national organizations—American Public Health Association and American Society on Aging. "I also try to do volunteer work. At the present time, I serve on the advisory council for a home health agency and the county health department."

Johnson's advice for a prospective nurse entrepreneur (male or female)? "Be very clear about what you consider to be your expertise and focus on that which you do well. Clients expect *expert* work and if you try to do too much, you can potentially run into problems."

Clifford Jordan, RN, EdD, FAAN, is a male nurse who has achieved national recognition. His sixteen-page curriculum vitae lists an impressive background that includes eighty-one papers and twenty-six published articles. Dr. Jordan, who is married to a nurse educator, agreed to share his ideas and beliefs as they relate to his own career: "My decision to enter and have a career in nursing was deliberate. It was not an alternative to medicine. I never wanted to be a physician. I have been a nurse for many years, and I have had, now have, and expect to continue to have fulfillment through nursing. I've touched all the bases. I have been a staff nurse, head nurse, supervisor, associate director, and director of nursing. I changed career goals at that point and became a nurse educator, where I achieved full professorship in a prestigious university (University of Pennsylvania) and its equally prestigious school of nursing. Currently, I hold the position of executive director of the Association of Operating Room Nurses.

"As a man in nursing I am often asked if I am discriminated against. I know there is discrimination against men in nursing, and that there are also real and psychological problems with the profession's and the public's acceptance of men in a 'women's profession.' I have known at least covert discrimination, perhaps not directed toward me personally, but rather as one of a class in the profession. I have achieved great success and recognition and have committed myself to helping young men and women to enter a field of health care that offers so much to enrich one's own life. I believe my success in nursing is directly linked to my qualifications, my manifest love of nursing, and my commitment to nursing.

"The public image of the nurse is changing. Nursing is more and more acknowledged as an autonomous health profession. Opportunities for careers in nursing are almost unlimited. The woman's movement (I prefer the term 'human movement') is liberating both women and men and that is helping those in nursing and those who will enter. The message is, 'it's OK to express emotions, it's OK to care, and both men and women can express that through nursing.'

"Nursing as a career provides economic security and an array of intangible benefits that can give those who enter full opportunity for self-actualization and fulfillment while they make a contribution to society that is unmatched by that of any of the other health professions. It has been a good life for me, one I intend to continue. I see no limits for those men who are qualified, aspire to national prominence, success, and making it to the top."

NURSE PRACTITIONER—TODAY'S PIONEER

Since 1965, when a demonstration project at University of Colorado first used the term nurse practitioner, things have not quite been the same for nursing. The concept of a nurse who functions as a primary health care provider is very exciting. Nurse practitioners work in an expanded role or in the role of the general practitioner of years ago. Defenders say that nurses are finally able to use the skills for which they've been trained. Detractors say that role is too much like the practice of medicine.

There's also controversy as to whether the nurse practitioner concept is even a new one. In 1925, Myra Breckinridge began the Frontier Nursing Service in a rural area of Kentucky. Famous for their midwifery service that brought nurses by horseback to patients' bedsides, the frontier nurses have now expanded their practice to include general family care. The program has been well received by the communities it serves and has obtained considerable funding over the years.

Nurse practitioners in the Frontier Nursing Service, and elsewhere, function independently or autonomously. Although working within established medical protocol, the nurse practitioner is the first person in the health care system to see and evaluate the patient. She is the one who establishes a plan of treatment and provides the continuity of care that each patient requires. It is within her province to counsel patients and refer them to other members of the health team (including physicians) as needed.

Nurse practitioners have additional knowledge and skills in areas that were once considered to be solely in the doctor's domain. But, first and foremost, they are nurses and are more concerned with the patient as a person than as a medical problem. So a nurse practitioner would not only take a medical history, do a physical examination, order diagnostic tests, and treat the patient's immediate problem. She would also assess the patient's psychosocial status and direct an overall health plan that would include prevention of disease and disability.

It is generally accepted that nurse practitioners can handle the majority of child and adult health problems with less cost and better care to the consumer than other providers. Physicians, as highly trained specialists, are the best providers of complex medical care but are over-trained for much of the work they now do.

A problem is that some physicians are threatened, professionally and economically, by the nurse practitioner role. In some areas, the established medical organizations have successfully lobbied against changes in the nurse practice acts that would legalize independent practice for nurse practitioners. Many physicians prefer hiring physician assistants, since their role is legally under the physician's jurisdiction.

In 1983, the District of Columbia was the first United States jurisdiction to pass legislation granting nurses clinical privileges (including admitting privileges) and staff membership. Since then other states have introduced legislation expanding nursing's scope of practice. Despite such legislative advances, nurses still face obstacles to independent practice through the regulatory process and other activities initiated by the medical profession.

Another problem is that of third-party payment. The Rural Health Clinics Act of 1977 paved the way for future revisions in third-party reimbursement for nurse practitioners. It enabled nurse practitioners to be reimbursed under Medicare and Medicaid for the services they provided in certified rural health clinics. The bill provided for direct third-party reimbursement in underserved areas, without requiring an accompanying physician's signature, as long as the nurse practitioner services were authorized under state legislation. There is still considerable variation in the type of reimbursement that third-party payers offer for nurse practitioner services. As of January 1986, 26 states had passed legislation concerning insurance reimbursement for nursing services. Some states allow for third-party reimbursement of nurse practitioners as one of many types of nursing services. Others have policies that focus solely on nurse practitioners.

Where does the nurse practitioner learn the additional skills that are required for her job? Educational programs are usually on the master's level although some programs award certificates at the completion of a prescribed course of study. The National League for Nursing believes that the nurse practitioner should hold a master's degree in nursing in order to ensure competence and quality care.

What is it like being a nurse practitioner today? There is great variety within this nursing model and it is impossible to delve into all the variations. But meeting a few of these professionals might give you an idea of how exciting this concept is.

Nurse-Midwives

Nurse-midwifery is not a new specialty, since the first school was started in 1931. However, it is enjoying a new wave of popularity and has been a model for many other nursing groups.

There are 3,000 certified nurse-midwives in the United States. To show the recent growth of this specialty, in 1970 the American College of Nurse Midwives had 550 members—in 1986, there were 2,700 members. Since 1980, the College has been certifying new nurse-midwives at a rate of 250 per year. In addition, in 1975, only 0.9 percent of all births were attended by certified nurse-midwives—in 1985, that figure had risen to 2.7 percent, according to the National Center of Health Statistics.

The practice of nurse-midwifery is legal in every state. Nurse-midwives practice in hospitals, birth centers, health maintenance organizations, public health departments, private practices, and clinics. They handle normal, uncomplicated pregnancies of which 85 percent are delivered in hospitals and 11 percent in birth centers. Earlier in this book I followed nurse-midwife Jan Hammond's management of one patient's labor and delivery (Chapter 1).

In addition to providing care to the pregnant woman and her newborn child, the nurse-midwife provides gynecological checkups, including physical examinations, Pap tests for cervical cancer, and breast examinations. The nurse-midwife will help the woman select a method of birth control and will refer the patient to a physician should there be a need for further medical evaluation.

The emphasis of the nurse-midwife's practice is on teaching and prevention of disease. In her day-to-day role, this means offering childbirth education classes and nutrition counseling. During labor, the nurse-midwife monitors the mother and fetus for complications and is supportive and eliminates uncomfortable and dehumanizing procedures. The nurse-midwife's philosophy is that pregnancy is generally a normal process but that it has the potential for complications. There is a necessity, therefore, for a physician to be in close contact with the nurse-midwife, but in an independent relationship.

The American College of Nurse Midwives (ACNM) is the professional organization that sets the standards for quality care and provides guidelines and accreditation for educational programs. There are twenty-five educational programs in the United States that are accredited or have preaccreditation status with the ACNM. According to this organization, the average full-time salary of certified nurse-midwives in 1986 was $30,936.

The future of nurse-midwifery appears to be very bright. One reason is the official endorsement of the American College of Obstetrics and Gynecologists, which states that a nurse-midwife, under the direction of an obstetrician in a hospital, may assume "complete management of the uncomplicated pregnant woman." A more important reason is that nurse-midwives provide warm, competent, attentive care at lower cost than do obstetricians.

Kathryn Kerrigan, a nurse-midwife who works in the family planning and women's health care clinics of the San Diego Department of Health Services, foresees increased acceptance and use of nurse practitioners in all health areas. Kerrigan's present position involves working one or two clinic sessions per day at the Health Department. She sees an average of fifteen to twenty patients at each session; does physical assessments, including gynecologic examinations; and is actively involved in teaching and counseling clients on the various types of contraceptive methods available to them. She is the only nurse-midwife on staff, so she also acts as a consultant to medical and nursing staff at the Department of Health Services.

Working in this type of out-patient community clinic is quite different from Kerrigan's previous position as a staff nurse-midwife in a large hospital, but she prefers this setting because of the greater opportunity for patient teaching. Kerrigan has found that women often feel freer to discuss personal problems—particularly those related to sex—with a female nurse-midwife rather than with a male obstetrician.

Before she attended the one-year primary-care nurse practitioner program at the University of California, San Diego, Kerrigan worked as a medical-surgical nurse at a community hospital and as a public health nurse, first for the New York City Health Department and then the San Diego County Department of Health Services. Kerrigan received her basic nursing education in a diploma program, then obtained a BSN at Boston College, and an MPH at San Diego State University.

The best part of her present position? "Knowing that I can make a unique contribution to patient care." Kerrigan continues: "Women in today's society are limiting their families to two or three children. Some women are delaying child bearing until educational and career goals have been achieved. These women are sophisticated and demand a more personalized type of obstetrical care. Many are seeking female health care providers who can relate to their special concerns.

"It is very satisfying to be able to help a couple experience a safe and satisfying birth experience by providing medical expertise along with emotional support. Being able to share in a special and possibly once-in-a-lifetime experience is a privilege.

"Caring for women from other cultures can be especially satisfying. Women from third-world countries have traditionally had female birth attendants. Many have had home births and are unaccustomed to and frightened by our modern technology. They need someone who can be mother, friend, and medical expert. The nurse-midwife can play all of these roles.

"I once delivered a young Vietnamese girl who was having her first baby. She spoke very little English and had only been in the United States for a short period of time. There were several family members in her room during labor. My communication with the family was limited, as I speak no Vietnamese. When I started coaching the girl to push her baby out, the family got down on their knees and began to pray. I was very touched by this sight. I can recall thinking how fortunate this girl was to have people praying for her and for her baby."

In order to be successful, Kerrigan feels that a nurse-midwife needs to be "a self-starter ... an achiever ... a risk taker ... and a person who can function under pressure."

Family Nurse Practitioner

Jacquelyn Dippert is a certified family nurse practitioner who works with her physician husband in a rural general practice in Eden, New York. Dippert explains her work situation: "I have a variety of duties in my practice. In addition to seeing patients with minor illnesses, performing follow-up and periodic examinations, I see all obstetric/gynecology patients, do well-baby checkups, and do all health care teaching.

"I work an eight-hour day in the office, usually beginning at 9:00 or 10:00 a.m., except for one late day when work begins at 1:00 p.m. and ends at 8:00 p.m. My regularly scheduled patients are seen by appointment, and in between I see patients with minor illnesses. This may involve taking a history on a patient the doctor will need to see, suturing a minor laceration, or assisting with minor surgical procedures.

"Once a month, before or after hours, I may visit the local nursing home to see our patients. I also routinely make house calls on a few of our elderly patients, especially in the winter months.

"Then there are meetings to attend, usually in the morning, at either of the local hospitals. At this time, I also make informal visits to any of our patients who are being hospitalized."

Dippert comments on the positive and negative aspects of her role: "I enjoy the freedom to be able to spend as much time as I feel necessary with each patient. It's difficult sometimes to get the staff to understand and promote the concept of the nurse practitioner. It is fairly new in our area and therefore unfamiliar to them. As well as the nurse practitioner is accepted by the patients, it is slower in coming among the other members of the health team."

Dippert graduated from a diploma program, the Buffalo General Hospital School of Nursing, and from the Albany Medical College primary care nurse practitioner program. She has been an RN for twenty-four years and has worked in various health care settings, including medical-surgical, gynecology, operating room, and emergency room units in various hospitals and also in doctors' offices.

The qualities most important for a nurse practitioner? "I think she has to be a caring, sincere individual who is a good listener and gets along well with people. Having a good sense of humor can be an asset. A nurse practitioner must also know her limits and keep within them.

"I would advise any nursing student interested in this type of career to gain a variety of nursing experiences before entering nurse practitioner school. I would also suggest that they observe a nurse practitioner in her health care setting in order to see the reality of the position before falling for the concept. It's always helpful to be aware of the market for nurse practitioners in the area in which you intend to practice."

Other Nurse Practitioners

Gretchen Green works with two family physicians in a rural health center in Freedom, Maine. She feels that the best part of her role is diagnosing and treating very ill patients. "There is a constant challenge to learn more, increase my skills, and accept more responsibility, although my title will probably not change. There may be friction with other nurses or health personnel—since they are reluctant to accept the new role of nurse practitioner—but the job is an exciting one."

One nurse practitioner in the San Diego area works in a joint practice with a busy orthopedist. Her day-to-day role involves applying and removing casts, performing minor surgery, suturing cuts, counseling patients before and after surgery, and dispensing medication under the physician's supervision. She is also in attendance in the operating room during elective surgery and visits hospital patients on regular rounds, writing instructions on their charts when needed.

A pediatric nurse practitioner may work with children in clinics, doctors' offices, health departments, and group practices. In one health maintenance organization in San Diego, the pediatric nurse practitioner manages checkups for well babies and children, assesses and treats selected childhood illnesses (with referral to the pediatrician when necessary), and provides guidance and health teaching to parents.

The role of the mental health nurse practitioner is similar, in many ways, to that of the clinical specialist in psychiatric nursing. Additional duties may include emergency psychiatric treatment and carrying a private caseload that may involve individual or group therapy.

Some pioneering nurse practitioners manage private practices, although they may function under very shaky legal guidelines. Nurse practice acts differ from state to state and are beginning to allow nurse practitioners greater autonomy. The ranks of nurse practitioners are growing, and future success will depend a great deal on decisions regarding legal constraints and financial reimbursement.

Nurse Entrepreneurs

The dictionary defines an entrepreneur as "one who assumes the risk and management of business." Within the last few years, an increasing number of nurses have become entrepreneurs and have started their own businesses in such fields as psychotherapy, home health care, midwifery, as well as educational and consulting services (earlier in this chapter, Michael Johnson was highlighted as a male nurse entrepreneur). Not all who make such a career change are successful, but each nurse who does succeed makes it easier for the nurse who follows. Three nurse entrepreneurs—Vicki Nenner, Jeanne Shaw and Audrey Mickel—tell their stories.

When Vicki Nenner, RN, began Marvik Educational Services in 1984, she and her partner expected that 80 percent of their clientele would be from hospitals and 20 percent from businesses. As it turned out, the exact opposite was the case—80 percent of her clientele have come from the business community and 20 percent from hospitals. Nenner's San Diego business provides two services: continuing education for health professionals and health promotion to business employees. Specifically, she has given programs on stress management for people who run residential care programs; has given classes to help employees stop smoking; has offered blood pressure screening programs at work sites; and has taught proper back care to hotel employees. This last program is offered in English and Spanish and instructors use lesson plans and hand-outs developed by the company.

Ms. Nenner had a business associated (Marilyn McCartney, RN) for two years but now runs the service herself out of her home. She has 80 people she can call on to teach classes. Ninety percent are nurses and many have other jobs.

"I keep regular hours—usually 8:00 to 4:30—and have a computer, copying machine and all the other necessary equipment. I'm the decision maker in the operation and that's exciting. Everyday I wake up, I look forward to what the day may bring. There's great variety too. For example, we've offered first aid classes to hang gliding instructors at a local Air Sports Center. And we've gone to hospitals and given review classes in basic skills for nurses."

The disadvantages of owning her own business? "It can get lonesome sometimes since I don't have the social interaction that I enjoyed when I worked at the hospital. For that reason I value even more the networking that I've established. Almost without exception, nurses have been very supportive of what I'm doing.

"The other drawback is that it was difficult to get the business off the ground. It took three years to break even. I would suggest that if a person isn't willing to invest that time and the effort that is required, they should find some other way to practice nursing."

Certainly Ms. Nenner has had considerable experience as a nurse. She received a baccalaureate degree from Texas Woman's University and spent one year as an intensive care nurse at St. Thomas' Hospital in London (this is the hospital where the Nightingale School began—see Chapter 2). Following this experience, she spent five years as an Air Force nurse and worked in Japan during the Viet Nam War.

"I worked for 11 years as Director of Continuing Education at a large San Diego hospital and, in 1984, received my master's degree from the University of San Diego. It was at this point that I saw the possibilities of starting my own business since I didn't see any way I could advance by staying in the hospital setting. Our company was incorporated in 1984 but I didn't resign from my hospital position until 1985."

Vicki Nenner's resume testifies to her diversified career. Every year she teaches a one-week management course at Clemson University in South Carolina and she recently agreed to serve as an at-large board member for the California League for Nursing.

And the future? "I see nurses becoming more and more involved in entrepreneurial activities. We have much to offer the public but are often frustrated creatively in institutional settings. This is a natural progression for nursing and I think it's great!"

Jeanne Shaw, RN, is a psychotherapist in an independent group practice in Atlanta, Georgia. She sees about 25 clients privately each week and also leads a two hour group therapy session. Seven therapists are equal partners in the practice, which is called Alliance for Counseling and Therapeutic Services, but Shaw is the only RN (one member is a social worker, the other five are clinical psychologists). The group owns the building in which they work and, all things considered, Shaw feels it's an ideal set-up.

"I'm my own boss although the partnership is a cooperative endeavor. I set my own fees, decide on the times I see patients and determine which patients I want to see."

Ms. Shaw received her baccalaureate and master's degree from Emory University. Before deciding on a career as a therapist, she worked in a hospital emergency room, a nursing home, and for Planned Parenthood. After receiving her master's degree in 1976, Shaw's faculty advisor in psychiatric/mental health nursing invited her to join the group practice.

"That nurse is presently out of the city, and is no longer in the practice; we've had some organizational changes since then. I've recently completed my dissertation for a PhD in Clinical Psychology through the external degree program at the Fielding Institute in Santa Barbara, California. Although the degree will allow me to sit for the psychology licensing exam and ultimately receive third party reimbursement, I plan to keep my identity as the nurse in the group. Many people are not intimidated by a nurse as they might be with other health professionals. They'll say, 'I don't need a shrink but I'll talk to a nurse.' I think we're seen as client advocates (with a specialized knowledge which includes ruling out medical conditions manifesting as emotional problems, and vice versa)."

Ms. Shaw suggests that if a nurse wants to start a business, it's necessary to do some homework.

"First, I think you should examine closely if being an entrepreneur would feel right for you. Some people want the security of working for someone else. Next, you should have a saleable skill that you enjoy and are good at. My specialty, for example, is sex and marital therapy and there are about 75 physicians, psychologists and nurses in Atlanta who refer patients to me."

"As far as getting the organization underway, I would suggest you seek out a number of competent people who have successfully started a business and study how they implemented their practice both with successes and failures. Then find yourself a good accountant and make sure you have enough money or credit to see you through the first lean years."

Ms. Shaw concludes, "You should use your nurse networking system for referrals and support. Visibility can be achieved by offering free programs to colleges and making yourself available to speak to professional and community organizations. Finally, you'll need a 'cuddle group'. That's what I call a group of peers who'll support and nourish you, both when things are not going well, and when they are going well."

Audrey Mickel, a nurse therapist practicing in San Francisco, has a unique business. She offers psychotherapy to about 20 clients per week using the special technique of imagery and self-management to heal various illnesses (imagery is a therapeutic tool used to treat various physical illnesses using imaginative thought). In addition, Ms. Mickel works as a consultant to government, private industry and other health programs. She gave assistance, for example, to the national job corps program in improving their health system and training their personnel. Nurse Mickel also frequently teaches at the University of Utah and gives seminars in guided imagery and healing to various organizations.

Her educational background includes graduation from a diploma program, BS in nursing from University of Virginia as well as masters and doctorate degrees in clinical psychology from the Professional School of Psychology in San Francisco.

Nurse Mickel receives most of her psychotherapy referrals from physicians and nurse practitioners. Marketing for the consulting and teaching side of her business comes mostly by word-of-mouth.

"Being an entrepreneur allows tremendous freedom and independence. Some weeks I may work 60 hours and other weeks it's less. I can usually schedule appointments to suit my convenience. Of course having the freedom to do what you choose and when you choose can be scary since you're the one that's determining the direction of the business."

Admittedly, Ms. Mickel's practice of nursing steps outside what some may consider the traditional boundaries of the health care system. However, she feels that this is the wave of the future.

"I think that nurses will be the ones to turn around health care in this country and will have the greatest impact on society."

TOMORROW'S CHALLENGE

General Trends

"With regard to nursing's future, I believe there really is a great deal to look forward to, although it will continue to be an uphill fight. Much depends on extraneous factors, which have a tremendous impact on nurse training and nurse practice but which nursing cannot control: for example, the role of the federal government in the delivery of health services, state budgetary restraints, changing health care technology, and the aging of the population."

These words belong to Sheila Patricia Burke, MPA, RN, who is staff director for Senate Minority Leader Robert Dole and works with many influential politicians.

Burke continues, "I would guess that we would see an increase in the use of nurses and services provided in noninstitutional practice sites: for example, homebased health care and ambulatory clinic care.

"Our recent experience suggests that nurses might begin to replace the old general practitioner of the prespecialization days in the health care system. This trend began in the early 1970s when the federal government decided to train nurses to deliver health care in areas where there were MD shortages. That was the beginning of nursing's involvement in primary care. The Rural Health Clinic Act, passed in the late seventies, was a further step in this direction.

"Licensure laws and payment systems are likely to encourage growth in independence for nurses, but narrowly so. Nurse practitioners and clinicians are more likely to be recognized through licensure laws and reimbursement systems as 'independent' providers than are hospital-based nurses. There will, however, be continued resistance from many payors to pay for those services not identified as traditional 'medical services.'"

Ms. Burke has an important position in the federal government, so her opinions are highly regarded. Other nurses are well known in the political arena. Forty-four nurses have been elected as state representatives and other nurses have had prominent positions within the

Department of Health and Human Services, or have been selected as White House fellows. From 1981 to 1985, Carolyne Davis, PhD, RN, FAAN was director of the Health Care Financing Administration, the agency responsible for Medicare and Medicaid. As patient advocates and promoters of quality care, nurses are challenging systems and organizations for the best interests of the profession and the nation's health.

Besides increased political involvement, what are some other trends that can be expected for nursing? Certainly there's room for more practitioners at all levels. Specifically, more nurses will probably be needed in geriatrics and critical care areas, but as Burke suggests, there will also be a need for more community nurses as expensive hospital care is replaced by cheaper free-standing clinics, hospice services, and home health agencies.

Federal budget cutting is a double-edged sword for nursing. While scholarships dry up and some agencies have to close their doors, lower-cost personnel (nurse practitioners) may be substituted for higher-cost personnel (primary physicians). This is seen as a positive step for nursing.

Expansion of health education is also good news, since this is an area that the profession has always promoted and has always accepted responsibility for providing. Past presidential administrations have tried to hold down health care costs for consumers by spending money for research, sponsoring Medicare and Medicaid, and giving financial incentives to health maintenance organizations. Recent budgetary restraints, however, have jeopardized many health and welfare programs.

The operative word for controlling health care costs for some politicians has been "competition." As government resources shrink, the private sector is taking over in the areas of research and health care. Proprietary hospitals (those owned by private corporations) are proving to be financially successful. Increasingly, doctors and nurses will have to be concerned not only with clinical expertise but also with business management. Nurse entrepreneurs are the newest pioneers in this resurgence of free enterprise as they carve out their own health and business ventures.

Technology

Can you imagine a robot folding sheets in the hospital's laundry room? How about a machine that would take samples of patients' blood or one that would get them out of bed on the first day after surgery? These and other so-called advances have been predicted by some scientists.

Increased technology is already a reality in critical care areas, as doctors and nurses analyze a patient's condition by observing dots and lines on an electronic monitoring machine. But will the use of computers and data processing make a nurse's life easier—from a management standpoint—or just take her further away from direct patient care?

Some feel that technology has become too important in health care today. Patients are overtreated, because the equipment is readily available (and has to be paid for). But who is there to hold the shaking hand or comfort the crying child?

As much as things change (and nurse specialization—with increasing skills—will continue), they remain the same: there's no substitute for the human connection. The caring and professional skills of a good nurse will always count as much as increased technological advances. Tomorrow's nurse will be held accountable in both areas.

Women and Nursing—New Images

When I was a nursing student, an instructor taught us how to write nursing notes in patients' charts: "Always use the word 'seem' or 'appear' when describing a patient's condition. For example, say, 'The patient appears to have stopped breathing,' not 'The patient stopped breathing.'" Presumably it was a legal question. If we said, "The patient stopped breathing," it would be making a diagnosis and that was something that only a doctor could do. Today nurses say, "The patient stopped breathing." They make other judgments as well and are held accountable for these judgments.

As nurses have taken on more and more responsibility, they expect recognition for the excellent care they provide. They expect recognition in the form of higher salaries and a better position within the health care system. Partly because of the spirit of feminism, partly because of increased education and greater technical responsibilities, nurses today want respect for the work that they do.

That's the heart of the matter and it's been a struggle for many years. But there are strong signs that nurses are finally being perceived as full-fledged professional members of the health care team.

The Nursing View

If Florence Nightingale were alive today, she would probably not be surprised by the continuing power struggles between physicians and nurses. She would undoubtedly be pleased to see the greater independence of today's nurse but might be overwhelmed by the many different specialties in which nurses have become involved.

Today, there are nurses who express disillusionment, frustration and, yes, anger at the stresses that they face daily. Some have left the profession all together and that's a sad occasion for everyone. But the majority of nurses today are convinced that their profession is unique and valuable. They feel that they can make a difference in patients' lives and would never consider another profession.

Dyanne Affonso, PhD, RN, is Associate Professor, School of Nursing at University of California, San Francisco. Ms. Affonso, the recipient of many honors and awards, has been called a nursing visionary and feels that now, more than ever, nurses need a collaborative spirit to make an impact on the nation. "Although this is a time of upheaval for nursing, it's also an exciting time filled with opportunity. The discipline of nursing—with its human element of care—will remain relevant no matter what other changes occur in the health care system."

Nursing will always need caring, competent, farsighted practitioners. What will be *your* role in the future of nursing?

APPENDIX

Additional Sources
of Information

INFORMATION ON EDUCATIONAL PROGRAMS

The **National League for Nursing** (10 Columbus Circle, New York, NY 10019) publishes numerous pamphlets about nursing education. The following booklets, updated yearly, give general descriptions of programs and list all accredited programs in each category: *Practical Nursing Career* (publication number 38-1328), *Associate Degree Education for Nursing* (publication number 23-1309), *Education for Nursing: The Diploma Way* (publication number 16-1314), *Baccalaureate Education in Nursing: Key to a Professional Career in Nursing* (publication number 15-1311), *Master's Education in Nursing: Route to Opportunities in Contemporary Nursing* (publication number 15-1312), and *Doctoral Programs in Nursing* (publication number 15-1448).

The NLN also publishes yearly listings of *State-Approved Schools of Nursing: RN* that lists all programs by state, with a separate section listing baccalaureate programs for RNs only. These and other NLN publications are listed in the yearly Publications Catalog, which is available upon request.

The **American Nurses' Association** (2420 Pershing Road, Kansas City, MO 64108) publishes *A Case for Baccalaureate Preparation in Nursing* (publication number NE-6), for prospective nurses and *Enrolling in a Baccalaureate Program in Nursing* (publication number NE-9), which describes the process of choosing and applying to baccalaureate programs.

For further information on external degree programs (available in New York and California) contact:

> The University of the State of New York
> The State Education Department
> Regents External Degree Program
> Cultural Education Center
> Albany, NY 12230

> California's Statewide Nursing Program
> California State University
> Domingues Hills
> 1000 E. Victoria Street
> Carson, CA 90747

Other sources of information include:

Barron's Profiles of American Colleges (Barron's Education Series, Inc., 113 Crossways Park Drive, Woodbury, NY 11797)

Cass, James, and Max Birnbaus, *Comparative Guide to American Colleges* (Harper & Row, 10 East 53 St., New York, NY 10022)

Lovejoy's College Guide (Simon & Schuster, 1230 Avenue of the Americas, New York, NY 10020)

Questions and Answers about Teenage Volunteer Services in Health Care Institutions (American Hospital Association, 4444 West Ferdinand, Chicago, IL 60624)

Gourman, Jack, *The Gourman Report—A Rating of Undergraduate Programs in American and International Universities* (National Education Standards, 624 South Grand Ave., Los Angeles, CA 90017)

INFORMATION ON FINANCIAL ASSISTANCE

Keeslar, Oreon, *Financial Aides for Higher Education* (William C. Brown Company, 2460 Kerper Blvd., Dubuque, IA 52001)

"Need A Lift?" (The American Legion, Box 1055, Indianapolis, IN 46206; $1.00 prepaid)

Scholarships and Loans for Beginning Education in Nursing (National League for Nursing, publication number 41-410)

Scholarships and Loans for Nursing Education (National League for Nursing, publication number 41-1964)

OTHER ORGANIZATIONS

Following is a listing of nursing and nursing-related specialty and special-interest organizations. Contact specific organizations for detailed information about certification and advanced training requirements. Organizations whose names are followed by an asterisk (*) are members of the National Federation of Specialty Nursing Organizations.

Alpha Tau Delta National Fraternity for Professional Nurses, 14631 No. 2nd Drive, Phoenix, AZ 85023

American Academy of Ambulatory Nursing Administration, N. Woodbury Road, Box 56, Pitman, NJ 08071

American Academy of Nurse Practitioners, 179 Princeton Blvd., Lowell, MA 01851

American Assembly for Men in Nursing, c/o College of Nursing, Rush University, 600 S. Paulina, 474-H, Chicago, IL 60612

American Association of Critical Care Nurses, One Civic Plaza, Newport Beach, CA 92660*

American Association of Nurse Anesthetists, 216 Higgins Road, Park Ridge, IL 60068*

American Association of Nurse Attorneys, Inc., P.O. Box 5564, Washington, DC 20016

American Association of Nursing Assistants, 145 East 84 Street, New York, NY 10028

American Association of Neuroscience Nurses, 218 N. Jefferson, Suite 204, Chicago, IL 60606

American Association of Occupational Health Nurses, 50 Lenox Pointe, Atlanta, GA 30324

American Association of Spinal Cord Injury Nurses, 432 Park Avenue South, New York, NY 10016

American Cancer Society, 90 Park Avenue, New York, NY 10016

American College of Nurse-Midwives, 1522 K Street, Suite 1120, Washington, DC 20005*

American Heart Association, 7320 Greenville Avenue, Dallas, TX 72531

American Holistic Nurses' Association, 205 St. Louis Street, Suite 506, Springfield, MO 65806

American Hospital Association, 840 N. Lake Shore Drive, Chicago, IL 60611

American Indian/Alaska Native Nurses Association, Inc., P.O. Box 3908, Lawrence, KS 66040

American Nephrology Nurses' Association, Box 56, North Woodbury Road, Pitman, NJ 08071*

American Nurses' Association, 2420 Pershing Road, Kansas City, MO 64108*

American Nurses Foundation, 2420 Pershing Road, Kansas City, MO 64108

American Organization of Nurse Executives, 840 N. Lake Shore Drive, Chicago, IL 60611

American Public Health Association, 1015 15th Street, NW, Washington, DC 20005*

American Radiological Nurses Association, c/o Elaine Deutsch, 502 Forest Court, Carrboro, NC 27510

American Society for Nursing Service Administrators, American Hospital Association, 840 N. Lake Shore Drive, Chicago, IL 60611

American Society of Ophthalmic Registered Nurses, P.O. Box 3030, San Francisco, CA 94119*

American Society of Plastic and Reconstructive Surgical Nurses, Inc., N. Woodbury Road, Box 56, Pitman, NJ 08071

American Society of Postanesthesia Nurses (ASPAN), P.O. Box 11083, 2405 Westwood Avenue, Richmond, VA 23230

American Urological Association, Allied, 6845 Lake Shore Drive. P.O. Box 9397, Raytown, MO 64133*

Association for Practitioners in Infection Control, 23341 N. Milwaukee Avenue, Half Day, IL 60069*

Association for the Care of Children's Health, 3615 Wisconsin Avenue, NW, Washington, DC 20016

Association of Nurses Practicing Independently, Department NL, 21 Spruce Street, Dansville, NY 14437

Association of Operating Room Nurses, Inc., 10170 East Mississippi Avenue, Denver, CO 80231*

Association of Pediatric Oncology Nurses, c/o Lorraine Bivalec, Pacific Medical Center, P.O. Box 7999, San Francisco, CA 94120

Association of Rehabilitation Nurses, 2506 Gross Point Road, Evanston, IL 60201*

Canadian Nurses Association, 50 The Driveway, Ottowa, Ontario, Canada K2P1E2

Dermatology Nurses' Association, North Woodbury Road, Box 56, Pitman, NJ 08071

Emergency Department Nurses' Association, 666 North Lake Shore Drive, Suite 1131, Chicago, IL 60611*

Gay Nurses' Alliance, 44 St. Mark's Place, New York, NY 10003

International Association for Enterostomal Therapy, Inc., 506 N. Tustin Avenue, Suite 282, Santa Ana, CA 92705*

International Council of Nurses, P.O. Box 42, 1211, Geneva 20, Switzerland

International Flying Nurses' Association, 3 Heidi Avenue, Middletown, NY 10940

Licensed Practical Nurses and Technicians of New York, Inc., 233 West 49 Street, 8th Fl., New York, NY 10019

National Association for Practical Nurse Education and Service, Inc., 254 West 31 Street, New York, NY 10001

National Association of Hispanic Nurses, 4359 Stockdale, San Antonio, TX 78233

National Association of Nurse Recruiters, 111 E. Wacker Drive, Suite 600, Chicago, IL 60601

National Association of Orthopedic Nurses, Inc., North Woodbury Road, Box 56, Pitman, NJ 08071

National Association of Pediatric Nurse Associates and Practitioners, North Woodbury Road, Box 56, Pitman, NJ 08071

National Association of Physicians' Nurses, 3837 Plaza Drive, Fairfax, VA 22030

National Association of Quality Assurance Professional, Inc., Department NL, 1800 Pickwick Avenue, Glenview, IL 60025

National Association of School Nurses, Inc., 7706 John Hancock Lane, Dayton, OH 45459*

National Black Nurses' Association, Inc., P.O. Box 18358, Boston, MA 02118

National Federation for Specialty Nursing Organizations, P.O. Box 23836, L'Enfant Plaza, S.W., Washington, DC 20024

National Intravenous Therapy Association, 87 Blanchard Road, Suite 4, Cambridge, MA 02138*

National League for Nursing, 10 Columbus Circle, New York, NY 10019*

National Male Nurse Association, 23309 State Street, Saginaw, MI 48602

National Nurses' Society on Alcoholism, P.O. Box 7728, Indian Creek Branch, Shawnee Mission, KS 66207*

National Rural Primary Care Association, Box 1211, Waterville, ME 04901

National Student Nurses Association, 10 Columbus Circle, 23rd floor, New York, NY 10019

Nurse Consultants Association, 870 El Camino del Mar, San Francisco, CA 94121

Nurses Association of the American College of Obstetricians and Gynecologists, 600 Maryland Avenue, SW, Suite 200 East, Washington, DC 20025-2589*

Nurses Christian Fellowship, 233 Langdon Street, Madison, WI 53703

N-CAP (Nurses Coalition for Action in Politics), Suite 408, 1101 14 Street, NW Washington, DC 20005

Nurses Now, P.O. Box 5156, Pittsburgh, PA 15206

Nurses Organization of the Veterans Administration, 23341 N. Milwaukee Avenue, Half Day, IL 60069

Nurses in Transition, P.O. Box 14472, San Francisco, CA 94114

Nurses' House, Inc., 60 East 42nd Street, Room 1616, New York, NY 10165

Oncology Nursing Society, 701 Washington Road, Pittsburgh, PA 15228*

Otorhinolaryngology & Head/Neck Nurses, c/o Warren Otologic Group, 3893 East Market Street, Warren, OH 44484

Sigma Theta Tau, National Honor Society for Nursing, 1100 West Michigan Street, Indianapolis, IN 46223

SAIN (Society for Advancement in Nursing, Inc.), Cooper Station, Box 307, 11 Street and 4 Avenue, New York, NY 10003

Society for Parenteral & Enteral Nutrition (ASPEN), 1025 Vermont Avenue, NW, Suite 8110, Department N, 81, Washington, DC 20005

Society of Gastrointestinal Assistants, Inc., 211 East 43 Street, Suite 1601, New York, NY 10017

Society of Nursing History, Nursing Education Department, Box 150, Teacher's College, Columbia University, New York, NY 10027

TRAVEL AND MILITARY CAREERS

Contact the following organizations for detailed information.

Department of the Air Force, Headquarters, U.S. Air Force Recruiting Service (ATC), Randolph Air Force Base, TX 78150-5421

Department of the Army, Headquarters, U.S. Army Recruiting Command, Fort Sheridan, Il 60037-6000

Department of the Navy, Navy Recruiting Command, 4015 Wilson Boulevard, Arlington, VA 22203-1911

Peace Corps, 806 Connecticut Avenue, N.W., Washington, DC 20525

Project HOPE, Health Sciences Education Center, Carter Hall, Millwood, VA 22646

Sherut La'am Long-Term Programs, American Zionist Youth Foundation, 515 Park Avenue, New York, NY 10022-1144

The American National Red Cross, National Headquarters, 17 and D Streets, N.W., Washington, DC 20006

U.S. Public Health Service, Department of Health and Human Services, 5600 Fishers Lane, Rm 17-74, Rockville, MD 20757

World Health Organization, (Pan American Health Organization), 525 23 Street, N.W., Washington, DC 20037

STATE BOARDS OF NURSING

ALABAMA
Board of Nursing
Suite #203
500 East Blvd.
Montgomery, AL 36117

ALASKA
Board of Nursing
The Frontier Building
Suite 722
3601 C Street
Anchorage, AK 99503

ARIZONA
Board of Nursing
Suite 103
505 N. 19 Avenue,
Phoenix, AZ 85015

ARKANSAS
Board of Nursing
Suite 800
11236 S. University
Little Rock, AR 72204

CALIFORNIA
Board of Nursing
Room 406
1020 N. Street
Sacramento, CA 95814

COLORADO
Board of Nursing
Room 132
1525 Sherman Street
Denver, CO 80203

CONNECTICUT
Board of Examiners for
Nursing
150 Washington Street
Hartford, CT 06106

DELAWARE
Board of Nursing
Margaret O'Neill Building
P.O. Box 1401
Dover, DE 19901

DISTRICT OF COLUMBIA
Nurses Examining Board
614 H Street, N.W.
Washington, DC 20001

FLORIDA
Board of Nursing
Suite 504
111 E. Coastline Drive
Jacksonville, FL 32202

GEORGIA
Board of Nursing
166 Pryor Street, S.W.
Atlanta, GA 30303

GUAM
Nurses Examining Board
P.O. Box 2816
Agana, Guam 96910

HAWAII
Board of Nursing
P.O. Box 3469
Honolulu, HI 96801

IDAHO
Board of Nursing
Hall of Mirrors
700 W. State Street
Boise, ID 83720

ILLINOIS
Department of Registration and
  Education
320 W. Washington Street
Springfield, IL 62786

INDIANA
Board of Nursing
Health Professions Bureau
One American Square
Suite 1020, Box 827067
Indianapolis, IN 46282

IOWA
Board of Nursing
1223 E. Court
Des Moines, IA 50319

KANSAS
Board of Nursing
Landon State Office Building
Suite 551S
900 S.W. Jackson
Topeka, KS 66612

KENTUCKY
Board of Nursing
Suite 430
4010 Dupont Circle
Louisville, KY 40207

LOUISIANA
Board of Nursing
Room 907
150 Baronne Street
New Orleans, LA 70112

MAINE
Board of Nursing
295 Water Street
Augusta ME 04330

MARYLAND
Board of Examiners of Nurses
201 West Preston Street
Baltimore, MD 21201

MASSACHUSETTS
Board of Registration in
  Nursing
Room 1519
100 Cambridge street
Boston, MA 02202

MICHIGAN
Board of Nursing
P.O. Box 30018
611 W. Ottowa Street
Lansing, MI 48909

MINNESOTA
Board of Nursing
Room 108
2700 University Avenue W.
St. Paul, MN 55114

MISSISSIPPI
Board of Nursing
Suite 101
135 Bounds Street
Jackson, MS 39206

MISSOURI
Board of Nursing
3523 N. Ten Mile Drive
P.O. Box 656
Jefferson City, MO 65102

MONTANA
Board of Nursing
Department of Commerce
1424 9th Avenue
Helena, MT 59620

NEBRASKA
Board of Nursing
P.O. Box 95007
State House Station
Lincoln, NE 68509

NEVADA
Board of Nursing
Suite 116
1281 Terminal Way
Reno, NV 89502

NEW HAMPSHIRE
Board of Nursing Education
and Nursing Registration
105 Loudon Road
Concord, NH 03301

NEW JERSEY
Board of Nursing
Room 319
1100 Raymond Blvd.
Newark, NJ 07102

NEW MEXICO
Board of Nursing
4125 Carlisle N.E.
Albuquerque, NM 87108

NEW YORK
Board for Nursing
State Education Department
Cultural Education Center
Albany, NY 12230

NORTH CAROLINA
Board of Nursing
P.O. Box 2129
Raleigh, NC 27602

NORTH DAKOTA
Board of Nursing
Suite 504
919 South 7 Street
Bismarck, ND 58504

OHIO
Board of Nursing Education
and Nurse Registration
Room 509
65 South Front Street
Columbus, OH 43215

OKLAHOMA
Board of Nurse Registration
and Nursing Education
Suite 524
2915 N. Classed Boulevard
Oklahoma City, OK 73106

OREGON
Board of Nursing
Room 904
1400 S.W. 5th Avenue
Portland, OR 97201

PENNSYLVANIA
Board of Nursing
P.O. Box 2649
Harrisburg, PA 17105

RHODE ISLAND
Board of Nurse Registration
and Nursing Education
Canon Health Building
Room 104
75 Davis Street
Providence, RI 02908

SOUTH CAROLINA
Board of Nursing
Suite 102
1777 St. Julian Place
Columbia, SC 29204

SOUTH DAKOTA
Board of Nursing
Suite 205
304 S. Phillips Avenue
Sioux Falls, SD 57102

TENNESSEE
Board of Nursing
283 Plus Park Boulevard
Nashville, TN 37217

TEXAS
Board of Nurse Examiners
Building C, Suite 225
1300 E. Anderson Lane
Austin, TX 78752

UTAH
Board of Nursing
Herber M. Wells Building
160 E. 300 South
P.O. Box 45802
Salt Lake City, UT 84145

VERMONT
Board of Nursing
Redstone Building
26 Terrace Street
Montpelier, VT 05602

VIRGIN ISLANDS
Board of Nursing
P.O. Box 7309
Charlotte Amalie
St. Thomas, VI 00801

VIRGINIA
Board of Nursing
1601 Rolling Hills Drive
Richmond, VA 23229

WASHINGTON
Board of Nursing
Division of Professional
   Licensing
Box 9649
Olympia, WA 98504

WEST VIRGINIA
Board of Examiners for
   Registered Nurses
Room 309, Embleton Building
922 Quarrier Street
Charleston, WV 25301

WISCONSIN
Board of Nursing
1400 E. Washington Avenue
P.O. Box 8935
Madison, WI 53708

WYOMING
Board of Nursing
Barrett Building
2301 Central Avenue
Cheyenne, WY 82202

Separate State Boards of Practical Nursing

CALIFORNIA
Board of Vocational Nurse and
   Psychiatric Technician
   Examiners
1020 N Street
Sacramento, CA 95814

DISTRICT OF COLUMBIA
Practical Nurses Examining
   Board
614 H Street, N.W.
Washington, DC 20001

GEORGIA
Board of Licensed Practical
  Nurses
166 Pryor Street, S.W.
Atlanta, GA 30303

LOUISIANA
Board of Practical Nurse
  Examiners
Room 1408
150 Baronne Street
New Orleans, LA 70112

TEXAS
Board of Vocational Nurse
  Examiners
Building C, Suite 285
1300 E. Anderson Lane
Austin, TX 78752

WASHINGTON
Board of Practical Nurse
  Examiners
Division of Professional
  Licensing
P.O. Box 9649
Olympia, WA 98504

WEST VIRGINIA
Board of Examiners for Licensed
  Practical Nurses
Room 506, Embleton Building
922 Quarrier Street
Charleston, WV 25301

Glossary

Accreditation.   Certification that a school of nursing has requested evaluation and successfully met criteria established by the state board of registered nursing and/or the National League for Nursing.

ANA.   American Nurses' Association—the national professional organization for registered nurses.

Articulated nursing program.   The baccalaureate nursing program that a student attends after having received his or her first nursing educational experience through an AD or diploma program.

Basic (generic) nursing program.   The baccalaureate nursing program that a student attends as his or her first educational experience.

Body-image.   A person's perception of his or her body and its parts and the ability to adapt to them as they exist.

Catheter.   A hollow tube used to remove or add fluids to the body or a tube used to establish the patency of a body structure.

Certification.   One form of credentialing whereby the quality of nursing care for various expanded or specialty roles is controlled. Certification is developed and maintained by professional organizations, such as ANA, or by individual institutions. Certification does not have legal status as licensure does.

CNM. Certified nurse-midwife—a nurse who has met certification standards to practice as a nurse-midwife and to provide care throughout pregnancy and birth. CNMs' scope of practice is defined by state law and differs from state to state.

CPR. Cardiopulmonary resuscitation—a prescribed sequence of steps, including the establishment of a clear open airway and closed-chest heart massage, designed to reestablish normal breathing and circulation after a patient's heart stops.

Credentialing. The awarding of a certificate in recognition of meeting specified requirements and attaining a specific level of competence. There are three types of credentialing in nursing: granting of degrees, licensure, and certification.

Defibrillation. The application of electric current to the heart to treat irregular heart rhythms.

Endotracheal tube. A specially constructed tube that is passed through the upper respiratory passages into the trachea and used to assist the patient's respirations.

Epidemiology. The study of the occurrence and spread of disease in the population as a whole.

Expanded nursing role. Positions in nursing that incorporate activities formerly not part of nursing.

Holism. The theory that a human being is more than the various parts of his or her physical body. In a holistic approach, each person is seen as an integration of body, mind, and spirit. When one of these systems is out of balance, all systems will be affected. In a holistic practice the total person must receive treatment, regardless of the patient's initial complaint.

Immunization. Injections given to patients to prevent certain diseases.

Incontinence. The inability of a patient to voluntarily control bladder elimination, bowel elimination, or both.

Intake-output. Measurement of the total amount of fluid and other substances entering the body by ingestion or parenterally. Also the measurement of fluids leaving the body.

IV.   Intravenous (within the veins). *Intravenous infusion* is the administration of certain fluids into the veins for therapeutic purposes. If blood is given, the infusion is called a *transfusion*.

Kardex.   A file containing the written nursing care plan for each patient on a unit. It is available to all members of the nursing staff and is updated as needed.

Licensure.   A mechanism for controlling the quality of professional practice within each state. A nurse becomes licensed after graduating from a state-approved school of nursing, passing the state board examinations, and meeting other set requirements.

Medical center (health science center).   A large hospital, or group of hospitals, usually near a medical school.

Medical protocol.   An established outline or plan for carrying out medical treatment.

Mouth-to-mouth resuscitation.   A first-aid method of artificial respiration in which the rescuer places his or her mouth tightly over the patient's mouth and forces air into the lungs in a regular rhythm. The rescuer then allows for a period of passive expiration.

N-G tube.   Nasogastric tube—a catheter inserted through the nose and ending in the stomach.

NLN.   National League for Nursing—the national organization that accredits nursing education programs and whose membership includes health care agencies and both nurses and non-nurses interested in the improvement of health care.

Nurse Practice Act.   Each state's legal definition of what nurses may do.

Nursing diagnosis.   The nurse's interpretation of collected information that indicates those patient needs that can be affected by nursing care.

Nursing model.   A method of presenting curriculum and caring for patients that uses nursing care, rather than medical care, as the focus.

Nursing orders.   Actions, set down in writing, that the nurse takes to help accomplish the established goals of the patient.

Nursing plan.   The methods that a nurse devises to promote the patient's recovery.

Nursing process.   A means of solving nursing problems by the processes of assessment, planning, implementation, and evaluation. Since the mid-1960s, many schools of nursing have used this concept in teaching nursing principles.

Paraplegia.   Paralysis of the lower limbs.

Physician.   A person who is authorized by law to practice medicine.

Physician assistant (PA).   A member of the health care team, the PA works dependently under the supervision of a physician and provides a broad range of health services normally considered in the physician's domain.

Primary health care.   The patient's first contact with the health care system in any given episode of illness. This contact leads to a decision of what must be done to help resolve the patient's problem. Physicians, dentists, and psychiatrists have traditionally provided primary health care. Nurse practitioners are new providers of such care.

Primary nursing.   An organizational pattern for delivery of nursing care that focuses on total responsibility by the professional nurse for a patient over a twenty-four hour period.

Quadriplegia.   Paralysis affecting the four extremities of the body.

Reality shock.   The syndrome experienced by new graduates, particularly those working in hospital settings. A conflict arises when professional nursing goals are seen to differ from the goals of the employing institution. This term was first used in the book *Reality Shock* by Marlene Kramer.

Standing orders.   Orders written by the physician for the routine care of the patient.

State Board of Registered Nursing.   The agency in each state (the title may vary slightly) that exercises legal control over nursing schools, curricula for nursing, and licensure of individual nurses within that state. The majority of board members are nurses and are appointed by the governor. The board, headed by an executive director, works closely with the ANA and NLN.

Suction.   The removal of air or fluids by negative pressure.

Third-party payer.   A source, other than the patient, that pays all or part of health care costs.

Tube feedings. Liquid nourishment given through a nasogastric tube.

Venipuncture. The puncture of a vein for various purposes.

Vital signs. Determinations that indicate the functioning of the patient's vital processes. Includes the recording of temperature, pulse, respirations, and blood pressure.

INDEX

Abdellah, Faye G., 163
Academic background, and admission to nursing program, 63–64
ACT, as factor in admission to nursing program, 64
Acute illnesses, 92
Administrator. *See* Nursing administrator; Hospital administrator
Admission of patient to hospital, 14–17
Admission to nursing programs, 46, 47, 49, 50, 54, 58–59
Advantages of nursing career. *See* Nursing career, advantages of
Agency nurses, 87, 136–139
Aides. *See* Nursing assistants
Air Force Nurse Corps, 24, 159–160, 211
Alcohol rehabilitation unit, 136
American Academy of Nurses, 77
American Association of Nurse Anesthetists, 100, 207
American College of Nurse Midwives, 194, 208
American Hospital Association, 65, 66, 206
American Journal of Nursing, 26, 75, 78

American National Red Cross, 24, 163–164, 212
American Nurse, 75
American Nurses' Association, 205–206, 208
  definition of nursing, 28
  function, 75–76
  position on nursing education, 46
  when established, 26
Anesthetist. *See* Nurse anesthetist
Aptitudes for nursing career, 33–36
Army Nurse Corps, 24, 156–158, 211
Articulated baccalaureate program, 61–62
Assignment, method of. *See also* Nursing specialties
  primary nursing, 85–86, 118–120
  task-oriented nursing, 85, 103–106
  team nursing, 85
Associate degree program, 26, 41, 45–46, 47–49

Baccalaureate program, 26, 41, 45–46, 54–58
Barton, Clara, 24
Basic baccalaureate program, 54–58, 61

Breckinridge, Myra, 191
Burke, Sheila Patricia, 201–202
Burn center, 111–114

Cancer nursing. *See* Oncology nursing
Cardiac rehabilitation units, 136
Career mobility, 73–74
Career planing
    choice of educational program,
        45–46, 61, 63–66
    choose place of employment, 69–71
    getting the facts, 38, 205–206
Certification, 88, 90, 100–101, 154
Childbirth. *See* Nurse-midwife;
    Obstetrical nursing
Children, nursing care of. *See* Pediatric
    nursing
Chronic illnesses, 92
Circulating nurse, 96
Clinical nurse specialist, 30, 40, 85,
    178–181
Clinics, public health, 149, 194
CNM. S*ee* Nurse-midwife
College education, trend for nursing,
    45–46
College entrance examinations, 64
Communications, as a career for
    nurses, 36–37, 181–183
Community nursing
    camp nurse, 140
    hospice nurse, 6–10
    nursing care in homes, 139
    occupational health nurse, 26, 39,
        40, 153–155
    office nurse, 39, 40, 141–143
    pharmaceutical sales, 140
    public health nurse, 25–26, 30–31,
        39, 40, 143–148, 149–150
    school nurse, 150–153
    visiting nurse, 31, 148–150
    wellness center, 140–141
Computers, use of in hospitals, 175,
    202
Consultant. *See* Nurse consultant
Continuing education
    as professional responsibility, 73
    to maintain license, 63, 73
Coronary care unit, 12, 110
Cost of health care, 123–125

Cost of nursing education, 47, 50, 54,
    58
Critical care nursing
    duties in intensive care unit,
        107–111, 112
Curricula
    associate degree program, 48–19
    baccalaureate program, 55–58
    diploma program, 50–54
    master's program, 59–61

Day care centers for elderly infirm, 139
Death, 6–10, 117, 119, 138–139
Diagnostic related groups (DRG)
    system, 37, 123
Dialysis nurse, 114–118
Diploma program, 41, 45, 49–54
Director of nursing service, 83,
    174–176
Dix, Dorothea, 24
Doctoral program for nurses, 41, 61
DRG system, *see* Diagnostic related
    groups

Educational mobility, 61–62, 73–75
Educational programs in nursing,
    45–62
    number programs and graduates, 45
    publications on, 205–206
    selecting a program, 45–46, 61,
        64–66
Elderly
    care of, 136–139
    need for nursing care, 42, 202
Emergency care, in the field, 10–14
Emergency clinics, 141–143
Emergency room nursing, 87–92
Employment agencies. *See* Agency
    nurses; Registry nurses
Enterostomal therapy, 120–123
Entrepreneur, *see* Nurse entrepreneur
External degree programs for nursing,
    62, 206

Family nurse practitioner, 195–196
Financial assistance, 206–207
Float nurses, 86–87
Frontier nurse clubs, 38
Future of nursing, 201–204

General duty nurse. *See* Staff nurse
Generalist, nurse, 93
Geriatric nursing, 42, 136–139
Goodrich, Annie, 26
Guidance counselor, as career advisor, 63–64

Handicapped, nursing care of, 131–136
Head nurse, 40, 83, 84
Health departments, and public health nurse, 30–31, 40, 149
Health education, 140–141
Health maintenance organization, 94–95, 123–124, 146
Henderson, Virginia, 28
Home health aides, 31–32, 145, 147
Home nursing care, 143–149
Hospice nurse, 6–10
Hospitals, 20, 81–84
    trend to shorter stays, 123–125
Hospital administrator, 82
Hospital nursing, 39, 40, 81–125
Hospital shifts, 86, 90

Imprint, 77
Independent practice associations (IPAs), 124
Industrial nurse. *See* Occupational health nurse
Infection control nurse, 83, 84
In-service education director, 83, 84
Intensive care nursing. *See* Critical-care nursing
Interests, personal, 33–34
International Council of Nurses, 76, 209
Internship programs for nurses, 72
IV team, 106

Job fairs, 69–70
Job mobility. *See* Career mobility
Jobs
    factors influencing choice of, 70–71
    how to find, 69–71
    salaries for, 40–41
Joint Commission on Accreditation of Healthcare Organizations, 65, 70, 82, 174
Journal of Enterostomal Therapy, 123

Journal of Practical Nursing, 78

Kardex, 15, 103

Licensed Practical Nurse, 78
Licensed practical nurse, 31, 136–139, 215–216
Licensed practical nurse program, 45, 46–47
Licensed vocational nurse. *See* Licensed practical nurse
Licensing of RNs, LPNs, 62–63

Mahoney, Mary, 25
Master's program for nurses, 41, 58–61, 192–193
Medial nursing, 14–18, 92–94, 179–181
Men in nursing, 6–10, 185–191
Midwife. *See* Nurse-midwife
Missionary nursing, 165–166
Mobile intensive care nurses, 88–91
Montag, Mildred, 26

National Association for Practical Nurse Education and Service, 78, 209
National Federation of Licensed Practical Nurses, 78
National Federation for Specialty Nursing Organizations, 77, 207–211
National League for Nursing
    accreditation of nursing schools, 65, 76
    position on nursing education, 46, 192–193
    publications, 76, 205
    when established, 26–27
National Male Nurse Association, 185, 188
National Student Nurse Association, 27, 76–77, 210
Navy Nurse Corps, 24, 158–159, 211
NCLEX, 62–63
Networking, 77, 175, 200
Nightingale, Florence, 21–23, 27–28, 203
Non-nurse college graduates, 74–75
Nurse anesthetist, 97–101
Nurse attorney, 176–178

Nurse consultant, 189–190, 200
Nurse educator, 40, 167–170
Nurse entrepreneur, 197–201
Nurse interests groups, 77–78, 207–211
Nurse-midwife, 1–6, 193–195
Nurse practice acts, 27, 192
Nurse practitioners, 29–30, 40,
　150–153, 191–197
Nurse registration act, first passed, 26
Nurse writer, *see* Communications
Nurses
　number, 39
　salaries of, 40–41
　where employed, 39
Nursing '88, 78
Nursing administrators, 40, 83–84,
　174–176
Nursing & Health Care, 76
Nursing assistants, 31–32
Nursing career
　advantages of, 36–38
　preparing for, 45–67
Nursing, definition of, 19, 27–29, 186
Nursing, history of, 19–27
Nursing homes, 39, 40, 136–139
Nursing organizations, 75–78, 207–211
Nursing Research, 78
Nursing schools, 45–66
Nursing shortage, 39, 41–43
Nursing specialties
　burn center, 110–114
　critical-care nursing, 107–110
　dialysis nursing, 114–118
　emergency room nursing, 87–92
　enterostomal therapy, 120–123
　geriatric nursing, 136–139
　medical nursing, 14–18, 92–94,
　　179–181
　nurse anesthetist, 97–101
　obstetrical nursing, 1–6, 101–103
　oncology nursing, 118–120
　pediatric nursing, 103–106
　psychiatric nursing, 127–131
　rehabilitation nursing, 131–136
　surgical nursing, 94–97, 143
Nursing staff in hospital, 82–84
Nursing supervisor, 40, 83, 84

Obstetrical nursing, 1–6, 101–103

Occupational health nurse, 26, 39, 40,
　153–155
Office nurse, 141–144
Ombudsman in hospital, 106
Oncology nursing, 118–120
Orderlies, 31–32
Orthopedic nursing, 94, 197

Paramedics, 11, 88–91
Patient advocate, nurse as, 117–119,
　202
Peace Corps, 160–162, 211
Pediatric nursing, 103–106
Physician-nurse relationship, 17–18,
　119, 187, 188
Political positions for nurses, 201–202
Pool nurses. *See* Agency nurses
Practical nurse. *See* Licensed practical
　nurse
Preferred provider organizations
　(PPOs), 124, 125
Private duty nurse, 39, 41, 83, 86
Professional nurse, 46
Project HOPE, 164–165, 211
Psychiatric nursing, 127–131
Public health nurse, 25–26, 30–31, 39,
　40, 144–150

Recovery room, 97, 99
Recruiters, 69–70
Red Cross nursing. *See* American
　National Red Cross
Registered nurse, 29. *See also* Nursing
　specialties
Registry nurses, 87
Rehabilitation nursing, 131–136
Religious orders and nursing, 20–21,
　23
Research nurse, 170–173
Richards, Linda, 24–25
RN, 78

Salaries, 40–41
SAT, as factor in admission to nursing
　programs, 64
Schedules, 86, 90
Schooling. *See* Educational programs in
　nursing
School nurse, 150–153

School of nursing, first, 23, 24
Scrub nurse, 96, 97
Selecting a nursing school, 64–66
Self-care, 140
Sigma Theta Tau, 77, 211
Staff nurse, 14–18, 40, 83, 84
State boards of nursing, 212–216
State Department, nursing opportunities with, 155–156
'Surgical day care centers, 143–144
Surgical nursing, 94–97, 143–144

Teachers, in nursing programs, 39, 40, 167–170
Technical nurse, 46
Technology and nursing, 202–203
Terminal illness. *See* Death
Third-party payment and nurse practitioners, 192
Traveling jobs
 military nursing, 155–160, 211
 missionary nursing, 165–166
 Peace Corps, 160–162, 211
 Project HOPE, 164–165, 211
 Red Cross nursing, 163–164, 212
 Sherut La'am long-term programs, 165–166, 212
 State Department, 155–156
 United States Public Health Service, 162–163, 212
 World Health Organization, 155, 212

Trends in nursing, 201–202

Uniform, nursing
 first American, 25
 in operating room, 96
Unions, 78–79
United States Public Health Service, 162–163, 212
Utilization review coordinator, 106

Visiting nurse, 31, 148–149
Vocational nurse. *See* Licensed practical nurse
Volunteer work, 66–67

Wald, Lillian, 25–26
Ward clerk, 83, 84
Wellness centers, 140–141
World Health Organization, 155, 212